BONDING BEFORE BIRTH:
A Guide to Becoming a Family

BONDING BEFORE BIRTH:
A Guide to Becoming a Family

LENI SCHWARTZ

SIGO PRESS
BOSTON

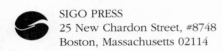

SIGO PRESS
25 New Chardon Street, #8748
Boston, Massachusetts 02114

Publisher and General Editor: Sisa Sternback

5/92

Library of Congress Cataloging-in-Publication Data

Schwartz, Leni.
    Bonding Before Birth: A Guide to Becoming a Family / Leni Schwartz.
        p.   cm.
    Includes bibliographical references and index.
    ISBN 1-879041-05-7 (cloth): $37.50. — ISBN 1-879041-04-9 (pbk.)
    : $16.95
    1. Pregnancy — Popular works.   I. Title.
    RG525.S3973   1991   91-19149
618.2'4—dc20   CIP

Printed in the United States of America, on acid-free paper.
∞

To my grandchildren
Jim, Emilou, Janey, Prinny

and their mother, my daughter Jay
and her grandchildren-to-be

CONTENTS

Forward

I am writing this as the mother of Adam, whose birth was transformed by our participation in a parenting group led by Leni Schwartz. My voice is heard in the group portion of this book as one of those affirming that there is a mighty life force at work during these nine months of pregnancy and birth, and we must not pass up the chance to explore the dimensions of it.

I am also writing as an anthropologist trained in the study of the modern American family and committed to the notion that there is no one right way. Some group somewhere has a different approach that works, and we might want to borrow some of their ideas.

Leni Schwartz has filled this book with wonderful ideas taken from many realms. Some originate from recent discoveries of science; some from other cultures; some from psychotherapy, the arts and design. Together they present an array of possibilities for shaping a unique path through the nine-month process of becoming parents.

This is not a book that makes the choices for you. Leni does not persuade you that home birth is best, for example. However, she does try to persuade you that the journey of pregnancy and birth is a unique time of growth and change that offers a chance to connect with the deepest self. It is an excellent time to ask questions, challenge assumptions, and affirm traditions.

This is as true for ment becoming fathers as it is for women becoming mothers. If we listen to men's voices in this book, we find that men have strong emotional reactions during this period but often feel left on the sidelines as observers of the heroine's journey. For those men who want to join in the process, this book provides the encouragement as well as specific examples of ways to do so.

Above all, the book provides men and women an array of choices and the courage to make them. It is a powerful gift.

Carol A. Richards, Ph.D.

Acknowledgments

So much of life's journey is represented in the creation of this book that it is impossible to list or even trace all those who have influenced it. So many have generously shared their time, their thinking and their hearts. Many advisors have become valued friends and many friends have been valued advisors. They have stimulated, challenged and nurtured me. In these pages I can name but a few who have played direct and indirect roles in helping me and this project along. To all those who have been an integral part of my life and to those with whom I have only had brief but significant contact, I am deeply grateful.

I am particularly indebted to Stanislov Grof, for it is out of his creative perception and research that my work evolved. His sustaining friendship and encouragement of the work I began was continually supportive. It was my friend, Jill Kneerim, who helped me initiate and focus this book. Without her generosity of time and spirit, professional clarity and belief in it, this book would never have come to be. She helped me find my own voice as I struggled to express myself in a new and unfamiliar form.

The ideas and encouragement of my doctoral committee started me on my journey. I wish to thank Rita Arditti, Norris Clement, Joan Halifax, Gay Luce, Lockwood Rush and Harold

Wise. They were challenging mentors. Harold Wise, joined by Richard Grossman, continued to influence my thinking as stimulating colleagues and close friends as we developed a model for "The Family Center" in New York. The support of the Benjamin Rosenthal Foundation made our year together possible. Joseph Campbell's vast knowledge of mythology and its relevance to the unfolding of life has been a source of inspiration and his friendship was a wellspring of support.

Many widened my perspective of this subject through the generous sharing of themselves and their work. In particular, I want to express gratitude to Suzanne Arms, Raven Long, Don Creevy, Sheila Kitzinger, Arthur Colman, Libby Colman, Rollo May, Jean Houston, Frederick Leboyer and Michel Odent.

I also wish to thank Suellen Miller, Ann Hubbell Maiden and Elizabeth Gilmore for critiquing the manuscript. I also appreciate the constructive suggestions offered by David Chamberlain, David Metcalf and Leah Morton for Chapter 2.

The experience of pregnant parents is at the heart of this book and I'd like to express my gratitude to each member of the Birth Workshops for their active participation, and to Maryallen Gessart and Charles Goodrich for their involvement and assistance in leading groups.

To my publisher, Sisa Sternback and my editor, Mary Ellen Lipionka, I offer warm thanks for help in shaping this book with their thoughtful, enriching suggestions and through their personal experiences as parents. Mary Ellen lavished sensitive, intelligent, and tactful attention to editing. I am grateful to Margery Berra, Kimberly Sheasby and Kay Carlsen for their careful and patient typing and retyping of revisions.

John Baxter has been a source of loving support in sustaining me, and a teacher in sharing his craft as a writer. Jackie Doyle was a mentor through her insight into the nature of relationships and her experience in leading groups. Many other good friends have helped with love, encouragement and ideas. I give loving thanks to my grown children, Jay, Andy, and Nikki, with whom I share the remarkable experience of family.

I thank everyone from the bottom of my heart.

INTRODUCTION

"It is only with the heart that one can see rightly. What is essential is invisible to the eye," said the fox in Antoine de Sainte-Exupery's The Little Prince.

Birth is the primal event for each of us. Being born is the earliest and most profound emotional shock to our psyches and bodies and may establish response patterns for future transitions that will take place throughout our lives. Psychoanalysts since Freud and Rank, as well as many philosophers and poets from the East and West, have long been telling us this. Conception, development for nine months in the womb, birth, and the first few hours of life are our first and most elemental experiences; yet, until recently, we have given the least attention to this period in our analysis of individual psychological development.

In 1840, Samuel Taylor Coleridge wrote, "The history of man for nine months preceding his birth would, probably, be far more interesting and contain events of greater moment than all the three score and ten years that follow it." In the past decade, many researchers continue to collect data that bear out Coleridge's statement. Yet, how many of us know about this critical period of our development? Twenty years ago when I began my work in the field of pregnancy and birth, there was comparatively little information about or belief in the possibility of remembering one's own birth or one's experience in the womb. However, evidence of this kind of recall is now proliferating.

In the early 70s I organized groups for parents-to-be, believing it was crucial to lend them support through the complex emotional gyrations of pregnancy. There seemed too little attention paid to the psychological changes that take place for mothers- and fathers-to-be as they move through this significant life transition. In my explorations into the field, I was discovering the importance of creating a harmonious and supportive environment for the parents, and therefore the baby, as they move through the normal yet dramatic changes that occur during the course of pregnancy.

Psychiatrist James Herzog of Harvard Medical School even suggests that a new field—the "psychoembryology of parenthood"—be given emphasis and be integrated into studies of fetal embryology. With this term, Herzog also acknowledges the importance of the inner life of expectant mothers and fathers and the role these emotional inner events play in affecting the parents' ability to bring into being and to nurture a child.

It has become clear that the baby developing in its mother's womb is affected by her emotional equilibrium and lifestyle, as well as by the world outside its mother's body. What's happening to the mother and father, therefore, is happening to the baby inside its contained environment. New studies reveal that our individuality develops in the womb amidst all these influences—that we are born into the world with a personality, temperament, and even predilections toward the behavior that will make up our adult character.

In working with the parents-to-be of the early support groups I organized, the ideas I presented were viewed with skepticism. I received the flak any pioneering work attracts. In professional lectures and workshops about the environment of birth and the psychological aspects of pregnancy, I was asked, "Why do you think *anyone's* behavior will affect the developing fetus? Can you *prove* there is consciousness in the womb?" Intuitively, I knew these things were important from what I had experienced and read. I searched for scientific data to prove my point of view and presented the then-limited studies, as well as my experience with pregnancy support groups, in lectures and workshops across the United States and in Europe between 1971 and 1978. Out of my work grew a book, *The World of the Unborn,* originally published in 1980.

In the ten years since the publication of my first book, an ever-increasing amount of clinical and empirical evidence has extended and deepened our awareness of the importance of the quality of experience in the womb, the birth process, and the primal hours after birth. Scientific methods of gathering information about fetal life have also become increasingly sophisticated and each new discovery informs further research. A fascinating kaleidoscopic view of fetal existence is now available.

There is agreement among those working in the perinatal field (*perinatal* encompasses the period before and after birth) that the way we are nurtured in the womb and the way we experience life during this developmental period influence our physical and psychological health and the way we will lead our lives. This body of evidence compels us to reorient our thinking and to integrate this crucial information into practice, for children represent the future, indeed the survival, of a nation. Therefore, understanding the transitional period when the family takes form is at the center of our shared emotional and physical well being.

At the heart of this book is the unborn baby and the ways in which it is affected by the emotional life and daily rhythms of its parents, by the environment in which its mother lives, and by the circumstances of its birth. The moment of conception, the process of growing in our mother's womb, reacting to her hormones, digestion, smells, tastes, the air she breathes, her movements and emotions for nine formative months, and experiencing birth, are all part of our unconscious, affective memories—remaining as a rich array of symbols and sensory recollections to influence our lifelong behavior. We may act out of the trauma of birth for many years, as psychologists suggest. Birth is a basis of emotional response, although we may not be conscious of what we are trying to create, avoid, or recall.

For most of my life, I have been an artist and a designer. As an interior designer, I have been fascinated with planning living spaces. For many years, I collaborated with architects and clients in creating spaces: conference centers, residences, offices, banks, hotels, motels, restaurants, and hospitals. Gradually, I began to question my status as an "expert" to whom people willingly yielded the power to make decisions about the environments in which they worked, played, lived, made love and raised their children. Why didn't people trust their own intuition and sensibilities, I wondered? That was in the 1960s. To find the answer to my question, I found myself gravitating from the role of professional designer to that of explorer in the field of self-awareness. Starting with a course in environmental psychology, I initiated a program of personal study. The people with whom I studied were exciting and stimulating—some of them pioneers of the human potential movement of the 60s and 70s, who involved me in the humanistic and transpersonal psychology movement in its initial stages. I became immersed in the study of humanistic psychology and the various integrative therapies that were developing, and ultimately I began training as a therapist. It was a fertile time for integrating new ideas with the wisdom of the past. (*Transpersonal psychology* means a relationship with the universal beyond the ego level, an extension of the *interpersonal*—a relationship between you and me—and the *intrapersonal*—a relationship with me and me).

One may ask how an artist and designer moved from designing spaces to studying environmental psychology and investigating the environment of the womb. It has been a somewhat circuitous and serendipitous path.

In the late 1950s I designed the interiors of a very special project called *The Motel on the Mountain* outside of New York City, which was influenced by the principles of Japanese architecture and design. It became quite celebrated. I collaborated with Japanese architect Junzo Yoshimura, a remarkable man who became an important philosophic and spiritual mentor for me. In the course of our work together, we spent long twilight hours talking about the contrast between life in Japan and in the

United States, about families, about Buddhism. It was a significant experience for me in which I began to understand the importance of wedding philosophic principles with the esthetics of architectural harmoniously integrated space with the natural environment.

Some years before, I had a memorable experience—an intimation of what my future work would reach for. In 1952, my husband and our two small children, ages two and three-and-a-half, were traveling in Kyoto, Japan, and stayed at a traditional Japanese inn (a *ryokan*). Established in our room, which was devoid of western furniture, I sat on a fat cushion on the grass-matted (*tatami*) floor overlooking the inner courtyard garden. The padded tatami mats formed a satisfying three- by six-foot module. We were served tea by a charming kimono-clad hostess who bowed herself gracefully in and out. In a short time, I became aware that I felt remarkably serene. Despite the fact that we had traveled for some hours to reach Kyoto and we, and especially two young children, needed time to adjust, the harmony I felt was remarkably deep and pervasive. From where did it emanate?

For a rare moment it seemed the architectural environment—its proportions, its colors, its textures, the garden, the way the activity flowed in the room—felt just right. At the same time, I realized that for most of my life it had not been so. For once, I was not subconsciously reordering volumes, forms, lines, colors, or the movement from outside/inside. In that instant, I was aware that upon entering a new space, I regularly went through a subconscious process of realigning what I felt were uncomfortable proportions, shapes, and colors. In my mind's eye I might move the ceiling two feet higher, the windows further apart; I might adjust the entry, mix a little more orange into the red to relate the color scheme. I began to realize how much energy I expended making the environment harmonious for myself. Here in this traditional Japanese inn, all proportions, textures, and colors felt aesthetically right. It was a very special experience of the principle of the Golden Mean. The serenity I felt as a consequence allowed me much more time and inner ease to simply be where I was. This realization of the effect of simple aesthetic

serenity was one of the turning points that led me to the study
of environmental psychology.

In 1970 I entered an independent study Ph.D. program at
the Union Institute in Cincinnati, Ohio, with a project that
began with a broad environmental focus and then became dramatically focused on my concept of "the environment of birth".
This new emphasis in my life and in my work was strength-
ened by an experience whose meaning and ramifications I am
still in the process of understanding. It was the re-evocation of
my own birth, described in detail in Chapter I. The ability to
"recall" my own birth implied that our personalities are influenced very early in development, possibly even in the womb,
and that we remember our earliest experience in some as yet
unknown way.

Environment has become a catch-all for so many causes that
its simple meaning has been obscured, and therefore the term
"environmental psychology," as an extension of it, may seem
vague and confusing. It is simply the study of influences, conditions and circumstances that surround us and affect our development and the way we respond and react. As individuals and
in group and community interaction, we are constantly modify-
ing and manipulating our environment. We do it to acquire
physical and social space that suits our needs. It is also a biological commonplace that occurs all around us; all life is
engaged in interacting with its environment, affecting and being
affected by it. The changes we make in our environment are
sometimes conscious, sometimes unconscious; yet, we have
discovered that once we intervene, more intervention is usually
required. Ultimately, the changes we have made may irre-
vocably and irreversibly alter us chemically, biologically and
behaviorally.

Environment in the broadest holistic sense is what surrounds
and supports us and influences our growth, development and
behavior. It is:

- The complex web of biological, psychological, social, cultural, ecological and transpersonal context that affects who
  we are and who we become.

- The envelope we call our body, its form and shape and biochemistry, which receives the messages from the society beyond it.
- The body as it expresses who we are, how we feel, how we wish to be seen and experienced.
- Our culture and ecology, which influence and alter our bodies and minds.
- The mind as it organizes the sensory input our bodies receive from the external world.
- The language, dance, music, art, and personal creative expression we share.

It encompasses our myths, our fears, our feelings of love, our interactions with each other, our inherited and unique experiences as members of the human species, and our transitional passages in the life cycle—an unending spiral of complexities that we only partially perceive and that affect us at every moment.

During the many transitions we make in a day, we move in and out of many environments. Many of these transitions are mundane and ordinary: I wake up from a dream state, tumble out of bed, and move through the cooler air of the hallway into the bathroom. It is the first of many transitions through which I will pass in the course of the day. My mini-environments change and yet are interconnected, if only by my passing through them. I am fortunate in that many are chosen by me, are in fact extensions of myself that give particular definition to my life: my house, my car, my neighborhood, my favorite restaurant or market, the region where I choose to live. Other environments are less personal: the street, the office, the store, public transportation. Some may be constricting, ugly and exhausting; others harmonious, beautiful, nurturing. I cope with all of these more or less unconsciously. Yet, as part of my ordinary daily experience, they integrally affect the way I feel and behave.

Some environments are extraordinary, like Chartres Cathedral, or the Grand Canyon, or our very first environment—the womb. Some transitions are unique, momentous, unforgettable, like our very first transition—birth.

The development of a new human being in the extraordinary environment of the womb has become for me a primary example of the interconnectedness, interdependence, and interpenetration of all things. In that remarkably designed, bounded, and protected environment within our mother's body, we are connected to the outer world. Within it we pass through many subtle transitory stages to our birth—our exit to the world beyond—the first major transit of many in the life cycle. Each time we make a major transition in our lives, moving from a known experience to an unknown one, we may reflect the psychological quality of our first transition into the unknown. Our primal environment and transition to the world beyond the womb may indeed be the template for the later transitions. It seems essential, therefore, to create a harmonious environment for gestation in the womb and a gentle and nurturing transition for birth so that those experiences become positive foundations for one's future.

The original focus of my studies in environmental psychology, as artist and designer, was to discover how we develop our individual sensibilities, taste, and preferences, how we relate to particular colors, forms, volumes, materials, and how we consequently validate our intuitive choices. I wanted to know if people prosper in aesthetically harmonious environments. Within the relatively new discipline of environmental psychology, sociologists, geographers, anthropologists, psychologists, architects, and designers are examining the complex layers of environment and the way those layers interweave to shape human experience.

In a similar way, I began to consider our first environment, the womb and the process of birth, and the physiological and psychosocial layers that interweave to shape our development and future at this primal stage. In my explorations and studies, I became fascinated by what I learned about the world of the unborn child and intrigued by the psychological developmental changes that occur during pregnancy for the parents as well. I began to feel that before I could consider the architectural design of more nurturing physical environments for this transformational period, I needed to understand more fully how the emotional impact of anger and frustration and love and compassion create a psychological environment for the parents and affect the physiological, psychological, and spiritual dimensions of this important rite of passage for the unborn child.

Consequently, in the early 1970s, based on my growing understanding of the developmental implications of "the pregnant year," I organized pregnancy support groups for fathers- and mothers-to-be who wanted to explore their complex feelings during pregnancy as they moved into the unknown, and who had begun to make an emotional connection to their not-yet-born children. In a sense, they were engaging in a "prenatal bonding" ritual. Although couples could not yet hold and touch their babies, they could speak to them, fantasize about them, visualize them in the womb, and imagine how their lives were affecting the baby's development. They could prepare for the next stage by making the transition to familyhood on a gradual basis rather than in one sudden plunge after labor and delivery. Couples who had not yet conceived were included. These support groups had enormous value for those who participated.

I hope that this book, which is an outcome of my Ph.D. study, will serve parents-to-be, and that includes any unit of mother and child and any family configuration, their families, and all those supporting this crucial transition called birth: doctor, midwives, nurses, psychologists, counselors, childbirth educators, and other health professionals. Also, I hope it will be of interest to each of us who has had our own experience of being born.

In the following chapters, I describe my quest for answers to the psychosocial dimensions of birthing. In Chapter I, I discuss the contributions of the many psychological researchers that have provided us with insight into our earliest personal history. In Chapter II, I introduce some of the fascinating scientific information about the development of the human being growing in the womb, which has been accumulating in the last decades. This is followed in Chapter III by a review of the complex stages of psychological development that parents-to-be move through during the course of pregnancy. In Chapter IV, I describe my early attempts to develop parent support workshops, the organization of the groups, and the experiences we had together. Chapter V chronicles the birthing experiences of some of the couples of the group, Chapter VI the recollections and reflections of group members six years later. In Chapter VII, I suggest specific ways in which others might make such groups a reality in their own community. Finally, in Chapter VIII, I offer my vision of an aesthetically harmonious Family Center that would provide not only a physical environment in which babies would be born, but would also become a psychological support center for the emotional shifts prospective parents experience during the course of pregnancy—a center in which the family's medical and emotional needs would be met with the highest regard for the health and well-being of everyone.

Writing as an environmental psychologist, it is not my intention to argue the scientific/medical aspects of birth practices. I leave that to the many fine books in the field. I want to focus particular attention on the dimensions of the psychosocial and spiritual experience. Yet, for me, of course, it is all interrelated.

This book is not only about the important rite of passage we call birth, it is also about the opportunity birth provides for understanding other aspects of our life and for the integration of all our experience. For the process of birth has become for me a metaphor for how the universe is patterned, the part standing for the whole—the *ordinary* experience enabling us to perceive the *extraordinary* dimensions of life.

It seems crucially important to bestow honor and value to American family life by creating support systems for parents as they move through this important transition. In this way we invest in the health, well being, and creativity of future generations. We can start at conception to work towards a more harmonious and peaceful world in which to live.

PROLOGUE

It was the first meeting of one of my support workshops for pregnant couples. As parents-to-be moving through the complex changes of pregnancy, they were to meet once a week for four months to share what was happening. After preliminary discussion, we began with an exercise designed to create bonding between parents and their developing baby even before birth.

> All of you are here as partners in a joint venture...Your baby is included as a silent partner...Over the next few months, we're going to engage in a bonding ritual with the babies in a daily conscious way even before they are born... To focus on this threesome, I'd like you to dialogue with your baby in the womb...Even though you cannot hold your baby or touch it, you can talk to it, fantasize about it, and begin to make a gradual transition into parenthood instead of making a sudden plunge after birth...close your eyes...get into a comfortable position...Begin to meditate on yourselves as a couple...and as a family...on two becoming three...Pay attention to your breathing and the flow of your partner's breathing as it enters your body...as it fills your heart, moves through the body, through your arms and legs and out again into the room, exhaling your breath out and inhaling it in again, adjusting the rhythm of your breathing to that of your partner's...And again inhale,

> be aware of your environment...focus on moving your
> breath through your body into your heart and into the heart
> of your baby....

No one in the room stirred, eyes were closed, fingers were
entwined. It appeared that each threesome was wrapped in
attentive meditation and visualization as they sat opposite each
other, knees touching.

> Allow your breath to flow freely from father to mother and
> child. Visualize the baby's environment inside the water-
> filled womb...Think about the baby's experience of its envi-
> ronment, its sense of you and the world beyond you. Think
> about what you are communicating right this minute to the
> responsive being who is forming in the womb, a baby that
> you have created. Think about yourself and what you feel
> as mother, as father, as a woman, as a man...Stay in touch
> with yourselves as a threesome, as a family...When you are
> ready, open your eyes slowly and gaze at each other. Take
> time to be with each other silently, and when you are
> ready, each of you individually write a dialogue with the
> baby.

There was stillness; there were no restless movements. Not
even Barbara stirred, despite the pressure of her full belly
pushed tight against her breasts. Jim's hands held hers, resting
on the shelf created by the swollen womb. Karin and Andy sat
on the floor, facing each other, no longer quite so erect, leaning
towards each other as they remained in meditation. Jim opened
his eyes and watched Barbara in her reverie, her eyes still
closed. Slowly he raised her left hand to his lips. She opened
her eyes to his touch, his head bent over his kiss. She smiled.

Everyone began to write. Twenty minutes later, we shared our
dialogues. The fathers began. Andy said:

> It's really hard to relate to you, since I can't see you or feel
> you. It's hard to believe in the reality of you living in the
> womb or even in my connection to you. Did I really have a
> part in conceiving you? My head tells me that's true, but my
> psyche is struggling to understand my part in it.

Jim wrote, "If I were you, kid, I'd want to get out of there."

Barbara was furious. It never occurred to her that her baby wasn't happy in the environment she was providing. She felt put down as Jim argued that nine months was a long time to be trapped in that space.

"What are you driving at in suggesting such a dialogue?" questioned Ed. "Do you really think we can affect the baby in the womb, by loving it, for instance? How can I influence the baby in my wife's belly?"

Although he admitted he was surprised by his sense of contact with the baby and had written three pages of dialogue, he insisted that he was not rationalizing those feelings away as he pressed for evidence. When I suggested that he did indeed affect his wife's emotions each day, which then directly influenced the baby's uterine existence, he laughingly denied that he had any sway over his wife.

"Anyway," said Ed, "what makes you think there is consciousness in the womb?"

He had raised one of the most fundamental questions of the workshop.

1

WHAT IS THE EXPERIENCE OF BIRTH?

Life is a continuity which does not begin at birth; it is split up by birth. The result of this splitting up is prenatal amnesia, but there is also an unconscious persistent effort to reestablish the lost continuity by annulling the trauma of birth.

Search for the Beloved, Nandor Fodor,

Birth is not a beginning...the true beginning is at conception. Nor is birth an ending. It is more nearly a bridge between two stages of life, and although the bridge is not a long one, a child crosses it slowly, so that his body may be ready when he steps off at the far end.

Life Before Birth, Ashley Montagu

As I began to seek answers to my questions about the experience of birth, I poured through the literature in the field and attended classes, lectures, and workshops. In the course of my explorations, in the fall of 1970 I attended a lecture in Silver Springs, Maryland, by Dr. Stanislav Grof, a renowned psychia-

choanalyst in Czechoslovakia, Dr. Grof had been involved in research at the Psychiatric Research Center in Prague in the area of altered states of consciousness. Since 1967 he has been working in the United States. During his talk, he spoke of psychological tools that, properly used, could enable one to study psychic material buried in the deepest layers of the unconscious that are usually inaccessible.

His theoretical framework for understanding the levels and dimensions of consciousness was derived from his analysis of material culled from three thousand patient sessions, conducted over the course of twenty years. During these sessions, all of his patients moved through similar levels of experience, although not always proceeding in the same order, and always through the psychological levels of their experience of birth, childhood, adulthood. Then, says Grof,

> They moved spontaneously into other experiential realms—levels that have been described through the millennia as occurring in various schools of mystical traditions, temple mysteries and rites of passage in many ancient and pre-technological cultures of the world. However, the most common, as well as the most important, of these phenomena were experiences of death and rebirth, followed by feelings of cosmic unity.

Without doubt, one of the major categories of these experiences observed by Grof is connected to the first and possibly most traumatic event of our lives: birth. Several times, in the course of long-term psychotherapy with Dr. Grof, most patients experienced a reenactment of the unexpectedly traumatic nature of the birth process: insistent pulsation of the womb's contractions, compressing sensations of the squeeze through the narrow opening, cranial pressure, rough handling by attendants and the profound shock of the sudden expulsion into the extrauterine world. Subjects frequently assumed postures and moved in complex sequences that resembled those of a baby at various stages of delivery. Grof, and many other therapists who have now developed a wide range of techniques that evoke powerful sensations seemingly related to the birth process, found that most participants later recounted the experience in incredulous language; it seems to be universally difficult to accept the idea of such preverbal memory. Yet, paradoxically, subjects remain convinced that they have experienced reenactments of their births.

Unavailable in the early 1970s when I began my explorations, data is now accumulating indicating that adults not only recover birth memories through various psychological therapies, but also that children of two and three speak quite spontaneously of life in the womb and of their birth experience. Linda Mathison of Seattle, Washington, has gathered many of these stories. These children remembering the womb describe the womb as "dark, crowded, like a big bowl of water or being in a pond." They speak of "liking the cord on me." Recalling their birth they say it was light after coming through the tunnel, and cold; "it was too tight;" "the light is too bright;" "it felt like a headache."

Dr. Grof's early observations suggested to him that the memory of our own birth may lie within each of us and can, under the right conditions, be evoked and "reexperienced." Extremely stimulated by the implications of his findings, I approached Dr. Grof after his talk and asked if we could meet again to discuss his research. We met the next day. I learned of the three research programs he was supervising as chief of psychiatric research at the Maryland Psychiatric Research Institute in Baltimore. Intrigued by the possibility that I might be able to reexperience my own birth, I volunteered for a project that was intended to study the experience of artists, writers, theologians, and psychologists. Through these various programs, Grof was continuing his long-term process of mapping the levels of the human unconscious. His recent books present his integrative transpersonal philosophy, clinical approach, and findings.

Working with Dr. Grof seemed to me a very special opportunity. Like most of us, I was searching for ways of understanding and expressing the core of self that is uniquely me. For me, explorative therapy with Grof promised to be a powerful way of reaching these deeper hidden levels.

A date was set for my first session. The afternoon before the scheduled session, I toured the research center and met Dr. Grof's colleagues. Grof and I then sat and talked about what I might expect. He suggested that I choose some favorite music from the record library that would evoke a range of emotional responses. During the session, he preferred to keep verbal communication to a minimum so that conversation would not intrude on my experience. He reviewed the nature of the states of consciousness that the experience might produce. He asked questions: How was I feeling? Was there anything in particular that I was concerned about? We talked about my personal history and about the issues I was confronting in the life transition through which I was moving. We discussed my longings and fears and expectations and the wide swings of elation and depression that I had been experiencing recently—not unlike the emotional ups and downs of the pregnant state. Indeed, I was pregnant with a new self. My three children were grown and off on their own, a new career was developing for me, and my relationship with my husband was changing. I was in a very new stage of my life.

Jung speaks of this period as a time of "individuation;" Maslow discusses "the movement towards self-actualization." I was committed to the idea that growth is an ongoing process and that self-knowledge is an essential part of one's creative unfolding. That summer I had traveled in Europe on my own, doing research for my doctorate. For the first time in twenty years, I was without family for an extended time. I recall turning around constantly to see where they were. During that summer, I had many symbolic birth dreams. According to the widely understood theories of dream symbology, these images represent the experience of birth: images of traveling on boats and trains, passing through tunnels, moving out of caves into the light, losing my clothes, finding new shoes. These symbolic birth dreams were encouraging me to break out of old patterns, to let go of the secure place, to journey into the unknown to allow a rebirth. How often we choose to cling to the known, the familiar, to the seemingly secure, unwilling to leave our childhood, a bad relationship, an unrewarding job.

Grof inquired about my dreams and fantasies of the past few days. We talked about letting go. Would I be able to let go during the experience? Surrender to the hidden parts of my unconscious? I wasn't certain. It was quite possible that by controlling my feelings, not allowing them to flood through me, I would resist the experience.

As we talked, I felt increasingly more at ease. Grof was professional, warm, impressively intelligent. He inspired confidence. I left this briefing session reassured and with positive feelings of anticipation.

The next day, I arrived at the center and was met by Grof at the appointed time. We talked together in the room that I had been shown the day before. It felt familiar—a pleasant room furnished with couches and chairs and attractive paintings. I felt refreshed by a long night's sleep and open to the experience that was about to begin. I had been observing my dreams during the preceding weeks, noting the feelings that were aroused.

I sat down on the couch, while Grof put on a record from the group that I had selected the day before. After putting on the earphones that Dr. Grof handed me, I stretched out on the couch and listened to the music. I began to breathe deeply under his guidance. The music was contemplative, calming. Gradually, it relaxed me. He gently guided me into deeper and deeper breathing. I recalled Grof's intellectual description as an important unifying and deepening element to the rebirthing sessions. Thoughts came and went. Deeper and deeper I went. A period of abstract imagery began in which forms appeared and disappeared kaleidoscopically; sometimes they were free form, sometimes geometric. They spiraled, twisted, whirled. I was totally absorbed in the intertwining of three moving strands. I moved into what seemed to be my body and sensed its form, from the molecular to the cellular and skeletal structure. I was both inside and outside; outside observing my bodily processes, inside experiencing them as they occurred.

The spiraling form with which I identified moved into a dim, enveloping, cavernous space. I felt its boundaries. How long I remained there I do not know. Neither time or space had any meaning, everything was happening in unlimited dimension. My consciousness swelled and completely filled the space I was occupying. I began to move slowly into a long dark tunnel. The walls moved in and out rhythmically, soft moist tissue contracting and expanding in a pulsating motion. At the end of the tunnel was a translucent, cerulean blue light, layered with lavender and sea green, like the clear blue of the most beautiful spring day. I was suffused with feelings of excitement and pleasure.

Quite abruptly, without warning, everything changed. Unbearable pressure was exerted on my head and body. The pain I experienced was excruciating. Though I was being pushed from behind by some implacable force, no forward movement was possible. Instead, the soft walls closed in. All movement stopped. Suffocating, I was caught in a vise-like grip, suffocating, too tiny and powerless to fight the unseen force. In an anguished cry, a mixture of rage and fear, I heard myself calling out, "Help me, I'm too small, I can't breathe, I can't make it alone. Why have you abandoned me? Where are you? I need you!" For what seemed an unending time, I felt I would die—alone, abandoned, imprisoned in the dark airless cage. There was no exit. I couldn't go forward and I couldn't go back.

Then, as inexplicably as they had stopped, the movements started again. The pulsation was intense and rhythmic. The soft walls moved in and out again...opening and closing around me. On the couch, I actually began to struggle—thrashing about, whimpering, and often crying in pain. Grof moved closer, sitting beside me on the couch, stroking my arm gently to reassure me. He didn't speak or intrude. I was simply aware that he was there. As my physical struggle became more intense, he cradled my head against his side. He seemed to sense I wanted something firm to push against; it was quite true. Although I was exerting all my strength, I couldn't push hard enough.

Strains of music wafted through my consciousness. It suited what was happening to me. I didn't try to identify it. Once or twice, I recall, Grof whispered into my ear underneath the headphones, "It's O.K. Don't resist your feelings. Experience it fully, whatever it is." Reassured by his presence, I resumed the titanic battle.

After what seemed like endless time, quite suddenly the struggle ceased and I burst out of my prison into a circle of clear blue light. It was an agonizing expulsion, accompanied by intense pain in my head and neck. I gasped for breath.

I lay still, painfully aware of my breathing. I was free.

Exhausted, but free. I moved into a state of euphoria, feeling light and happy. For an undefined period, I was cradled by Grof, wanting nothing more than to be held. At moments, it seemed that I was not breathing at all. Everything was in stasis. I was a totally dependent being. Then I would become frightened and a whole other chain of emotions would begin in me...increasing sadness followed by tears, a sense of abandonment and despair...then the cycle would begin once again— struggle, pain, the sense of being caged—changing into a feeling of release, euphoria, peace, light. These sensations continued to play themselves out like my own personal movie inside my head, continuing for hours, reels and reels of images appearing and disappearing, unfolding in a series of changing scenes, characters and events. As the intensity of sensory experience abated, I was more able to take in the feeling that had been evoked. The incredible kaleidoscope of memories, of feelings and events remained with me for a long time in quite remarkable detail. Joy, sadness, glory and terror, the present and future were experienced as an incredible array of sequences parading through my mind and emotions. I have returned to it many times to unravel its extensive metaphor and meaning. My perceptions and attitudes shifted, creating a whole new lens through which to view my experience. Although my avenue of personal exploration might not be the way for everyone, it was fruitful for me in terms of understanding myself and my life, as well as providing me with insights into the work I chose to do.

The next day, Grof and I talked about my "birth" experience, the images and events and the feelings that had been evoked. It was like opening the floodgates—and was the first of many talks. Mostly, I wanted to sit quietly and contemplate the day's happenings and the emotions that were stirring within me. As I settled into the present, I found myself in a wondrous emotional state...everything freshly perceived, senses expanded. Later, surrounded by close, affectionate companions, I relished the tastes, smells, textures and visual beauty of dinner. The world seemed exquisite. Although I went to bed early, it was hours before I fell asleep.

The next morning, Grof and I met again to analyze the experience. My years of psychoanalysis and self-inquiry helped me to work with the powerful images and feelings that had come to the surface. Could it be that I reexperienced my birth, that I had symbolically moved through the birth canal and had been expelled from the womb? Could it possibly be that so many years after that event, I had brought to a conscious level the pre-verbal memory of my birth?

With these questions in mind, I decided to approach my mother as soon as possible for help in reconstructing the events of the day of my birth. Amazingly, I had never thought to ask her for any of these details before—as I'm sure is true for many of us.

In retrospect, it seemed quite remarkable to me that I had so clearly perceived my mother as my opponent during the "birth" experience, involved as we had been in a joint endeavor. What if there were a grain of truth in my perceptions? Had she "given up" during labor in the face of overwhelming obstacles? If so, for what reason had she abandoned me in the middle of the journey, leaving me to feel as if I had to perform the monumental task alone?

I later discovered that she in fact had been completely abandoned by her maternity nurse. When she arrived at the hospital in the early stages of labor, she had been walked up and down the halls according to the practice of the day, until the amniotic sac broke. She remembered that the doctor came to examine her about 10 A.M. and warned the nurse that when the bag of waters was broken, the baby would come fast. Those were the early days of hospital births with no analgesic drugs nor any real preparation for the experience. At about eleven o'clock, lunchtime for the private nurse, mother was put to bed in her private room, patted on the head as if she were a child and told by her private nurse to hold on tight until she and the doctor returned from their lunch hour. Her nurse warned her that the other floor nurses would not respond to her ring since she was in charge of a private nurse and it was she who would call the doctor. Alone and frightened, my mother lay rigid in her narrow hospital bed, tensing every muscle in her body in hopes that she could hold me back until they returned, terrified that I might be born as she lay there alone and unattended in that strange room. She was scared and in a lot of pain, she said. When the nurse returned an hour later, bringing the doctor with her, my mother relaxed her hold on me. She was taken to the delivery room. I was delivered twenty minutes later.

How long do those psychological traces remain with us to govern our responses? I realized in my own case it was for a long time. With surprise, I recognized that I often gave up when getting "stuck" in the middle of a large project, frozen by feelings of frustration and anger. With much effort, I would summon up all my strength and go at it again and usually break through. What amazed me was how repeatable this pattern was. Are these reactions imprinted on us and passed onto the generations that follow? Nightmares experienced when we are sleeping prove that we need not be conscious to experience fear and mental anguish. Do we each carry with us frightening, repressed memories of our own births? Psychological data indicates that we do. Does it matter? Is it important? I believe that it is of vital importance. Birth (like death) deserves an important place on the map of formative events in our consideration of human consciousness. Most of us, and certainly as counselors and therapists, can benefit from understanding the perinatal experience.

Twenty years ago when I began my work there was little information about birth memory; however, it is now proliferating. Psychologist Dr. David Chamberlain's book, *Babies Remember Birth*, (1988), brings these fascinating research findings to the public. In his practice as a hypnotherapist, he heard many "seeming birth memories." With the permission of his patients, he began to record, transcribe, and analyze them. Studying, researching, learning was a thirteen year adventure for him.

Perhaps the techniques now being developed by various therapies will give us the tools to bring our earliest memories to consciousness. It would be valuable for each of us to know about the circumstances of our first nine months in the womb, to become aware of the earliest influences that formed our personalities. Like the ancient Chinese, we might consider that our "birthdays" are marked from the time of conception.

Puzzling "accounts of memories of birth" have been quietly

reported since the 1890s but were confused and treated skepti-
cally, or were simply dismissed. More recently, however, prenatal memories are being evoked by many therapies such as
rebirthing, hypnotic regression, psychodrama, and holding and
breathing therapies, and recall is more readily accessible.

Other psychological techniques such as dream work, primal
therapy, waking fantasies, and water therapies have also been
evocative. Furthermore, during altered states of consciousness
and meditative states many people have reexperienced their
births. Yogic breathing and body therapy techniques like those
developed by Wilhelm Reich in the 30s have now been further
developed by others and also bring repressed memories to the
surface.

In the 70s, psychologist Elizabeth Fehr pioneered a therapy
which combined hypnotic regression and body movement to
create a rebirthing technique. Unfortunately Fehr died quite
young and was unable to carry her work further. Her methods,
however, influenced the late British psychotherapist R. D. Laing
in his work of the 1970s, and many others.

My own "rebirthing" under Fehr's guidance occurred several
years after my work with Grof. Fehr, a clinical psychologist, had
been recommended to me by Dr. Laing, who knew of my interest in the psychological consequences of birth. Fehr's method
had developed from observations of a difficult, inarticulate
patient. During the course of several therapy sessions, his con-
torted body posture suggested to her the possibility of a complicated birth experience. Pursuing that hunch over a period of
many months, she guided him through hypnotic regression,
which led him back to birth. The course of therapy released him
from his neurotic behavior. For Fehr, it created a new direction
for her clinical explorations.

Her means of releasing unconscious material was quite different from Grof's. For example, she used props, a thirty-foot foam
rubber "birth canal," two companions to form the uterine wall,
and a series of verbal directions to guide her patients. It was an
active and physical process. During my session, I was asked to
lie on my back with my knees up and my feet on the floor and
inch my way down "the birth canal." Two women lay close

beside me on the floor and moved along with me with rhythmic pressure representing uterine contractions. My physical and psychological responses corresponded to those I had displayed in the session with Grof. As before, I became immobilized close to the end of the "birth reenactment," stuck again as I had been during my actual birth. Along the way, and particularly at the point where I lay motionless, Fehr suggested quietly I could reshape my present experience and erase the old nonproductive, blocked memories. "It's all right," said she, sitting beside me, reassuring me, "I believe you had trouble in your birth at this particular point right before delivery. Do you know that is so? This time you can create a new way."

She touched me tenderly. Mustering all the energy I could, I got myself moving again. I began to feel empowered as I traveled the rest of the way with the help of my "womb" companions, the group members travelling beside me. It proved, once again, to be a release of my fear of getting stuck.

Psychologist Arthur Janov's primal therapy, also developed in the 1970s, encourages participants to fully express and confront their intrauterine memories and the physical pain of the birth shock. He utilizes techniques of breathing and vocalizing designed to break through body armor which Janov believes begins to form at birth in reaction to our first "primal" trauma.

Grof and his wife Christina have more recently developed a powerful deep yogic breathing in a system they have developed, called holotropic therapy. Like other systems, it releases unconscious material and facilitates movement through many traumatic events.

In a recent conference on perinatal issues that I attended, keynote speaker pediatrician Lee Salk discussed stress experienced by babies during birth. The stress, he feels, is somatized in particular organs as weaknesses which become sources for medical problems throughout life. He emphasized the need to be concerned with the physical and emotional vulnerability of this critical period. New data supports his concerns.

Therapists working with birth trauma feel that virtually all births are traumatic and lifelong reactive patterns can be set up as a result of the experience. Many believe, however, that recog-

nizing the importance of a harmonious pregnancy, and good
bonding at birth and in the first weeks after birth, will probably
alleviate the trauma and replace it with a positive imprint. It has
been demonstrated that a baby cuddled and bonded to its mother at birth will be able to weather future crises more readily. The
data now accumulating demonstrates the importance of repat-
terning the way we think about pregnancy and birth.

Consideration of birth as an important aspect of the study of
human psychology in the Western world is relatively recent, if
one recalls that it was in the 1920s that Sigmund Freud and his
disciple, Otto Rank, were debating its importance in psychoanalysis. Although it was Freud who said, "All anxiety goes back
originally to the anxiety of birth," and who suggested that the
pain of being born and the threat of suffocation during birth was
a basic model for the later attacks of fear, he did not pursue this
aspect of anxiety in his work. Real memories, wrote Freud, are
stored in the unconscious and continue to influence our behavior throughout our lives despite our ability to repress memories
on a conscious level. We "act out" those repressed memories
unconsciously in repetitive behavior until they are brought to
conscious awareness.

Rank, however, was deeply influenced by the idea of the anxiety of birth. It became a cornerstone of his work. *The Trauma
of Birth* outlines his theory, stressing the traumatic effect of the
separation of mother and child, which he called "the primal cas-
tration." We would now call it "lack of bonding." It was a radical
idea in 1924.

Rank emphasized the traumatic aspects of transition from the
peace and security of the womb to the harsh realities of
extrauterine life. "To be born is to be cast out of the Garden of
Eden," said Rank, "and there follows a continuous effort to
return to that lost paradise." "The primal anxiety" created by the
birth trauma, somehow "blots out the memory of the former
pleasurable state." Rank felt it was the first experience of repres-
sion and selective memory. Most of our childhood is required to
overcome the trauma and to reexperience the pleasure of the
womb. He also spoke of birth in terms of the hero's journey. As
we undergo a psychological as well as a physical transformation,

each of us is a hero at our birth. The primal anxiety that originates at birth is free-floating and may transfer itself to almost any source. As children, in games and fantasies we try to discharge the unreleased anxiety by acting it out again and again. Consciously and unconsciously, we seek catharsis. We try to recapture the rhythms and security of the womb as we rock in chairs, swing, are carried in planes and boats, float about in lakes and oceans, or seek the warm comfort of our baths and beds, in order to effect a cure.

It was Rank's idea, for example, that hide-and-seek games were in fact, an acting out process representing painful separation from mother and the relief and joy at finding her again. Rank's system of psychoanalysis based all psychological problems on the trauma of birth. Interestingly, his system was reported to be quite effective, requiring only four to eight months for treatment instead of the Freudian system, which took many years. Other psychotherapists and researchers through the years have come to share Rank's view of the power of the birth experience to affect later behavior. Sixty years later, we are witnessing a renewal of interest in Rank's ideas. New therapies are being developed to help us recognize and work through the effects of the birth trauma. Since the 1920s, important material in support of Rank's point of view has come from contemporary clinical work.

Birth memories were reported at the turn of the century, often by medical doctors working with patients under hypnosis, but the idea was scoffed at. It was not given serious attention as an area for research until forty or fifty years later. Research therapists, such as Grof, Chamberlain, and other clinical therapists, have repeatedly reported and described the occurrence of birth memories or "experiences" during their patient sessions. Unable to demonstrate literal "memory recall," they usually considered these experiences "allegorical birth fantasies." American psychoanalyst Nandor Fodor called them "organismic impression."

Dr. Carl Whitaker, an eminent psychiatrist and family therapist at the University of Wisconsin Medical School, said to me in the 70s:

> Back in the days when we were using intensive regression as a modality of psychotherapy, I went through the birth experience with many psychotics and many "normal" people. I was always too embarrassed to talk about these experiences because I felt that nobody except the patient and my colleagues at the clinic would believe that these people were really reexperiencing their own birth.

However, in spite of the otherworldly quality of these experiences, and the prevalence of symbolic and archetypal images, there is often striking agreement with the actual physical aspects of the subject's birth. In addition, details are often substantiated by parental accounts, such as my mother's.

The work of Grof and others in the 60s, 70s and 80s, has dramatically augmented our knowledge of birth trauma, leading scientists such as Carl Sagan, in his book *Broca's Brain,* to question exactly how much we do in fact remember of our perinatal experience and what the consequences of those memories, painful or otherwise, might be.

> We must ask why such recollections are possible—why, if the perinatal experience has produced enormous unhappiness, evolution has not selected out the negative psychological consequences....[The] answer might be that the pros outweigh the cons—perhaps the loss of a universe to which we are perfectly adjusted motivates us powerfully to change the world and improve the human circumstance. Perhaps that striving, questing aspect of the human spirit would be absent if it were not for the suffering of birth.

In the 1950s, Nandor Fodor in his book, *Search for the Beloved,* offered some of the insights that have contributed to present day thinking. He reported that many birth events were recalled by his patients: annoyance with bright lights used during postbirth surgery, memory of a cold environment, fear of loud noise. He spoke of chronic adult symptoms that were connected to early experiences.

Even Fodor was perplexed when he observed that patients appeared to be reliving their womb experience or birth in his presence, in his consulting room. He, like others, was skeptical, for there was no substantial data supporting the idea of memories or even a "real mind" operating at such an early stage in human development. However, intuition told him that there was telepathic communication between mother and the baby in utero in some way he could not explain scientifically.

A well-known hypnotic researcher and longtime obstetrician, Dr. David Cheek of San Francisco, has been using age-regression hypnosis for many years as a technique for releasing suppressed memories of birth trauma, which he feels is at the root of many medical symptoms of adult patients. Former president of the American Society for Clinical Hypnosis, Cheek also believes that patients are able to recall and reenact preverbal experience in a trance state.

Cheek and Ernest Rossi in their book *Mind-Body Therapy* discuss the concept of cellular memory. As early as six or seven weeks in utero, the baby has body chemicals in place that carry messages throughout its system. Rossi and Cheek contend that a baby after birth has the capacity to remember these messages (especially emotionally charged ones) after birth, and that the memories become imprinted. Cheek defines imprinting as "any emotional response that becomes fixed by the emotional or physiological stress with which it first appears." Bad imprinting repeats like a cassette on automatic. Obviously, some of these imprinted behaviors are neither desirable nor useful to us as adults. However, says Cheek, unlike animals, human beings can simulate the recreation of an event, and in the process can envision a more appropriate integration of the experience. In agreement with Fehr and others, Cheek contends that we may have the ability to alter this so-called imprinting and develop new behavior patterns.

The key to this process may lie in our ability to simulate, or reexperience, events such as our own birth. Yet, since it is virtually impossible to verify that a patient is recalling the actual events of his or her birth, the most one can say is that during the session the patient is experiencing the sensations of birth. Whether the therapeutically experienced birth resembles the actual historical birth cannot, of course, be proven. In his book, *Realms of the Human Unconscious,* Grof concurs that the authenticity of recapturing memories of womb and birth events is open to question. He has tried to remain as open-minded as possible about this "phenomena" and furthermore has tried to verify reported episodes by questioning the mother or other persons who were involved, as has Chamberlain. He stresses that he takes the precautions necessary to avoid contaminating the data. He reports that despite their reluctance to accept the idea of prenatal memory before their sessions, the psychologists and biologists who volunteered as subjects for his research programs were quite astonished at how authentic and convincing their experiences were. "The existence of such phenomena," says Grof, "was contrary to their present scientific beliefs."

In the 1970s I traveled to Paris to meet the poetic French obstetrician Frederick Leboyer, author of *Birth Without Violence.* His book was not yet published in the United States and he was in the process of editing his affecting film, *Birth.* I was much moved by his ideas and felt privileged to observe him delivering several babies in his clinic. In the last decade he had come to the conclusion that the love and care a child receives during labor and post-birth are decisive factors in alleviating the intensity of traumatic stress. Some years earlier while undergoing analysis, after twenty years of traditional obstetrical practice in Paris, Leboyer became painfully aware of the traumatic effects of his own birth. The development of his ideas and his now well-known and influential method (which he adamantly explains is not a method, but an attitude or a "protocol" for birth) emerged out of the reexperiences of his own thirty-hour biological labor in which he "felt" he was facing death. As a result of psychoanalysis and his intense study and practice of Buddhism in India and Europe, he became psychologically and philosophically more aware, compassionately identifying with the baby's titanic struggle into life. Out of this awareness have come three beautiful books and a film that describe his "nonviolent" approach to birth. His ideas were challenging and helped create change in both the parents' attitudes, and in the practices of the obstetrical profession. But the wholehearted embrace of new ideas comes about slowly, especially when the scientifically trained are asked to integrate love as part of a "medical" procedure.

Dr. Michel Odent and his colleagues in the maternity unit were much affected by Leboyer's book and film and have carried the work further by observing and listening sensitively to mothers during the course of pregnancy and birth. As a surgeon in the municipal hospital in Pithiviers, France, Odent was called into the maternity unit to handle obstetrical complications. In this way, he became increasingly involved with the birthing process. With the midwives, he collaborated in creating an environment in the hospital where birthing mothers could have the support and freedom to give birth according to their individual needs. "We were ready for it," he says. "But it was pregnant women who actually enabled us to understand Leboyer so quickly." They were aware that he was not talking about a technique but about an attitude change, an environment in which a loving entry into life could be facilitated. Odent is now working in England, applying his ideas of "primal health" to a physical form.

Not only is birth itself being considered in a new light, but there is significant research on the importance of the first hours after birth. It is a crucial time, a shared state of heightened consciousness for both mother and baby. Some suggest that postbirth physical contact is so integral a part of the birth process that it may be seen as the fourth stage of labor and should not be considered only as a part of the delivery process.

Psychological "imprinting" immediately after birth is relevant in this period. German ethologist Konrad Lorenz spoke of it as a "sensitive period"—a once in a lifetime opportunity for attachment that would never again be available. In his study of animal behavior in the 50s, he observed that a gosling becomes bonded for life to the first animal it had contact with after birth. The significance of the period immediately following birth for the emotional well-being of the baby has also been clearly shown by the pioneering work of Drs. Marshall Klaus and John Kennell at Case Western Reserve Medical School in Cleveland. It is part of nature's patterning. A baby is biochemically designed to communicate with its mother, as is a mother to bond with her newborn.

That process is innate and appears to be a sophisticated signaling system between mother and child. Films of mother-child interaction clearly demonstrate the instinctive "getting acquainted" process, the repetitive ritualistic pattern that we now refer to as "bonding." Intriguingly, most new mothers follow the same sequence in handling and caressing their naked newborns. As the mother strokes and fondles her baby she has carried for nine months, she is discovering on the outside the person she has known inside her body. Bonding immediately after birth and for a period of five hours or more enables mother and child to relax together intimately after the hard work of birthing.

Klaus believes that as the mother touches her baby, gazes into its eyes, soothes its naked body with skin overly sensitized by the experience of its birth, she is going through a ritual of "knowing" it to be hers. It is the first intuitive manifestation of maternal love and attachment outside the womb experience. "We think," said Klaus, "that when we put the body of a mother close to her baby, something is turned up in her genetic make-up." Odent states it in biochemical terms pointing out that in the first hour neither mother nor baby have eliminated the hormones secreted during birth that are essential to the attachment process. Some researchers suggest that these hormones are secreted early in fetal life to initiate attachment while the baby is developing in the womb. The Sufis speak of this in a different way: one must avert one's gaze from the eyes of the newborn until the baby has looked into the eyes of the mother, otherwise, it is interference in the natural order of life.

In the studies of Klaus and Kennell, women who were able to have immediate extended physical contact with their babies formed deeper attachments than mothers who were not permitted, because of hospital regulations, to perform the bonding ritual. Mothers need to be able to welcome their baby in their unique way. All animals exhibit this welcoming behavior. Newborns need the tender welcome and security of maternal touch. We know that babies that are not bonded may die— either an actual physical death or a psychological one and are forever in search of the missing bond. The "bonding" period has been well documented for animals by scientists like Lorenz and

Harlow, who discovered that brief periods of partial or complete separation after birth may drastically distort a mother animal's feeding and caring for her infant. It has also been documented that loving touch and gentle massage help a newborn gain weight more quickly. Loving touch is essential to physical and psychological growth. The baby has already been stimulated by touch in utero. It touches the soft fleshy walls of the womb, its own body, the umbilical cord, it sucks its fingers and even toes sometimes.

It is quite clear that the occurrences of the first few hours after birth determine the future development of the child. These primary hours are of utmost significance. In the first few hours after birth, a baby's body is adjusting to its separate existence. The newborn baby does this best next to the security of its mother's body—her rhythms, her smell, her touch, her voice, her breast. It is mutually rewarding for both mother and baby. If, for some medical reason, a mother cannot be with her newborn immediately after birth, it is possible to have the father or a motherly surrogate hold and touch the baby. The work of Marshall and Phyllis Klaus, which they are now continuing at Children's Hospital in Oakland, California, John Kennell, Lee Salk, T. Berry Brazelton, Frederick Leboyer, Michel Odent among many others, has forced a thorough review of perinatal practices and has caused many American hospitals to reconsider former routine procedures. One hopes the trauma of birth *is* lessening in this and other ways. Yet still much more needs to be done. These ideas are still not widely accepted, however, even now; many years after these principles have been demonstrated, change comes slowly.

The personal work I did with Grof in my rebirth experience had affected me profoundly, as did the research I read thereafter. My perceptions and attitudes shifted dramatically. I began to perceive new connections between events in my life and saw my own experiences as continuous and interrelated rather than mysterious and random. I realized that patterns of behavior repeated themselves when stimulated by deep traumas and emotional injuries as far back in one's personal history as the womb. Until brought to conscious awareness, confronted, and worked through, they would continue on automatic replay. My thinking also expanded to a deeper appreciation of the remarkable order and pattern in nature. Not only did I become more connected to my inner self but that self became more connected to everything beyond it. The concepts of continuity and harmony became guiding themes for me. It was through this personal journey that I came to be intensely interested in the circumstances surrounding pregnancy—the pregnant year and the environment of birth, what is now called by many the perinatal experience.

I came to understand that "birth" is not a single event but a process that begins at conception, is established at implantation, and embraces nine months in the womb, the momentous journey down the birth canal toward a separate existence, birth itself, and the subsequent postnatal bonding experience. In those first nine months and beyond, I believe, we experience the sense of oneness—an oceanic bliss—at the same time that we suffer the opposite sensations, earthbound discomforts caused by our mother's activities as she copes with the complex demands and the irksome stress of her daily life and by our father's daily life and temperament. It is our first intimation of the balance of opposites that exist in the world we will soon enter.

Listening to the Child Within

Lie on the floor, nestling close to each other.... Father, place your hand over the womb over your baby. Mother, place your hand over your partner's hand. Close your eyes. Still your mind by focusing on your breathing; take a deep breath and let it go. Allow your body to melt into the floor.

Breathe gently and deeply, inhale and exhale, feel your tension relax with each exhaled breath. Inhale and exhale; listen with your heart to your feelings and thoughts, to your inner dialogue. Pay attention to everything that is happening within you: become aware of the rhythm of your breathing, let it join the rhythm of your partner's breathing.... Sense the flow between you as a couple. Imagine yourself as a parent, as partners, as a family—one becoming two becoming three. Be aware of the life developing in the womb; sense the presence of your baby.

Allow your breath to flow from one to the other, and then to your baby, until you sense that all three are in rhythm with each other. Imagine your baby's environment inside its water-filled chamber. What is your baby experiencing? Listen! What is your baby communicating to you now? What does your baby need? Listen with all your being....

Say goodbye to your baby now. Begin to stir; become aware of the floor beneath you and the air around you. When you are ready, open your eyes, and with a soft unfocused gaze, look around you. Be aware of where you are and how you feel and slowly come back to this room.

2

NINE MONTHS OF CHANGE:
INFLUENCES IN THE WOMB ENVIRONMENT

For a long time, poets, mystics, and some scholars have intuited the importance of the prenatal period; however, only recently has medical science been able to systematically study the mystery of our beginnings, following its time-honored studies of the life cycles of other species and its inquiries into many other aspects of human biology and experience. The investigation is now aided by advanced technology of the scanning electron microscope, fiber optics and special lenses, ultrasound imaging and other measuring devices, time lapse photography and advanced laboratory techniques, which have provided tools to observe and measure the baby's responses in its womb environment. The studies of biochemists and neuroscientists have given us keys to further understanding, and medical observations in the care of *premature* babies have increased our knowledge of a baby's development from the sixth month *in utero* to term.

It is surprising to realize that embryology obstetrics, pediatrics and gynecology—those specialized branches of medicine that care for women and children—are only about seventy years old and that the field of fetology, devoted to the care and understanding of the baby from conception to birth, is only about thirty years old.

Of course, serious studies of fetal life have been made for many years, even before the discipline had a name. One of the early researchers in this field, Dr. Lester W. Sontag of the Fels Research Institute in Yellow Springs, Ohio, a contributor of important pioneering studies since the 1930s and 1940s, suggests poetically that one reason so little consideration has been given to behavior in the womb and the environmental factors that influence it may be our difficulty in accepting the idea that "the human psyche might know of its own coming." Far Eastern thought, with its belief in reincarnation, has accepted the idea of prenatal consciousness for centuries. Yet scientifically-oriented Western society has not dealt with the idea of consciousness or emotional awareness as a human being develops in the womb. According to Western thought, in previous times it was believed that a baby *in utero* could not feel, hear, see, taste, sense or remember. John Locke, in the seventeenth century, stated that a baby was a blank slate (*tabula rasa*). Researchers have now discovered quite a different picture.

The work of Dr. Stanislav Grof, as well as the works of many other pioneer researchers such as Candace Pert, Dr. Michele Clements, Dr. Alfred Tomatis, Dr. Henry Truby, Drs. William and Margaret Liley, and many others too numerous to mention, have made seminal contributions to this new field of inquiry. In Europe in the 1970s a new discipline of prenatal psychology evolved that embraces pre- and perinatal psychology, focusing on everything concerning the birth experience. It adds information to research from other fields. More recently, an International Congress of Pre- and Perinatal Psychology of North America has been established, meeting every other year to discuss recent findings in obstetrics, neurophysiology, anthropology, fetal psychology, and other allied subjects. Information, data and educational material are rapidly being disseminated from this new field in the human sciences.

Recent studies indicate that the baby in the womb senses and responds to its immediate environment to a greater extent than we had thought possible, and the womb is probably where our first learning takes place as our developing senses respond to our experience. Increasing evidence also shows that parents' life style and emotions and also external environmental factors are more important to an unborn baby's psychological development than was previously realized. In one sense, we are witnessing a resurgence of the old belief in the power of "maternal impressions" to affect the baby's development, although this resurgence is based on new scientific understanding rather than on superstition. It is now considered in terms of mediating influences, such as stress-induced hormones, new findings in neurophysiology, and other factors to explain what was previously inexplicable.

In this chapter, we will look at the wondrous development of the fetus in the womb in terms of its progressively more complicated behavior patterns as it moves toward human beingness and viability—life outside the womb on its own. Then we will examine some of the evidence that leads us to believe that psychological development in the womb may be more subject to external environmental factors than anyone considered until recently. It is not intended as an exhaustive scientific account but rather as an appreciation of the capacities of the infant in the womb in light of new theories and knowledge. A more comprehensive source is *Babies Remember Birth* by Dr. David Chamberlain, a book filled with scientific discoveries about fetal development, prenatal learning, newborn communication, and bonding.

The conception of a new human being, though an ordinary occurrence, seems an extraordinary miracle. The complex process of human development begins with the simple fertilization of the human egg. This process—conception—although simple, is remarkably dramatic.

At Tokyo's Toho University School of Medicine, Dr. Motoyuki Hayashi developed a way of filming the initiation of life. Using advanced instruments, time-lapse photography, and a culdoscope, he has filmed rabbits and monkeys as stand-ins for the human experience. He describes conception as a volcano erupting as the mother's ovary swells, ejects fluids and cells, and finally a mature egg. The egg then is moved through the fallopian tube into the uterus by finger-like projections called fimbria—a journey of five inches that takes from five to seven days. The several million sperm released by the father-to-be during intercourse make the swim upward of less than a foot into the fallopian tube to reach the egg. Swimming frantically, their black tails parallel, only a few of the strongest sperm competitors will reach the receptive egg in a race that takes anywhere from a few minutes to an hour. In a dance of life, the remaining sperm surround the egg on its journey through the fallopian tube. As they crash into the egg attempting to penetrate the egg's protective covering, they send it spinning counter-clockwise. Once a single sperm triumphs, others are prevented from entering by a chemical change. As the fertilized egg continues its journey to the womb, it develops into a blastocyst—a ball of cells. Within ten days, embedded in the wall of the womb, the rapid division and multiplication of cells continues—numbering several million. In this tiny bit of protoplasm, cells grow rapidly, and within them resides the basis for all the structure and organs that will form an intricate, complex human being at birth.

Is it possible that this powerful experience is recorded somewhere in the psyche?

In its well-lined, shock-absorbing uterine sac, which nature has so remarkably designed, the tiny organism will float and swim in a warm, watery world, warmer by one degree than its mother's body temperature. Within this dimly lit, humid container, connected to its mother and to the outside world, the unborn baby will have its first experiences of interacting with its environment. During its nine-month sojourn, as it rapidly develops in complexity into human form and capacity, it will begin to respond to its inner world and to the outer world beyond. Although well-protected within its mother's womb, contrary to earlier belief, it is a more permeable environment than we suspected, requiring sensitive nurturance and protection.

As we know, this fertilized egg contains all the genetic information necessary to produce a person at the end of its gestation in the womb. Within this tiny human organism, visible only through a magnifying lens, live the genes that it inherits from its parents. Yet it is the combination of the basic genetic endowment bestowed by its parents, the normal course of the baby's development in the womb, the influence of the mother's environment and lifestyle during pregnancy, and the circumstances of its birth and the bonding between mother and child thereafter that will create the unique qualities parents will observe in their newborn.

The question as to whether heredity or environment is more influential—the old nature versus nurture controversy—is now obsolete. Recent thinking affirms that the baby's genes and its environment work integrally together. Inherited genes, for example, may determine eye color, blood type, or one's potential height; however, diet, exercise, stress, and the baby's general health will influence whether or not that height will be attained. Just what, then, are the influences on the baby's development in the womb?

Until very recently, says biochemist Rene Dubos, it was customary to regard the nine months in the womb and newborn states as relatively unaffected by the external environment, except for instances where infection or other obvious threats existed. We now know, however, that variations in the womb environment, and the mother's lifestyle and external environment, can profoundly affect growth, development and even the personality of her child. A baby is affected by its mother's temperament, lifestyle, and her daily habits as she lives through each day. As she receives stimulation from her environment, she reacts and her child in her womb receives this stimulation through her body. The womb environment is affected. It is a form of "learning" that affects the unborn baby's growth and physical and psychological development. Her moods also affect her unborn, who responds differently when she is rushed or relaxed, tense or calm, happy or enraged. Her baby in the womb is affected directly, as it cannot escape the effects in its contained environment. Her baby's activity and heart rate shows a marked increase when she is emotionally disturbed and is quieter when she is at ease. How differentiated these mood tones are, as experienced by the baby, is being actively investigated. Being able to connect and communicate with her unborn child in a nurturing way can be an important positive biochemical component of womb existence.

Within the protective custody of its mother's body, the developing human being is experiencing the world even as it passes through its rapid developmental stages from embryo to fetus to newborn baby. Each stage of the unborn baby's development has its specific tasks and needs, and it is wise to be aware of them and respectful of nature as the ultimate designer. The unborn experiences the outer environment and even the nature of its culture through its mother's daily interactions in it, and also through its own interactions with the outside world (through the vibrations of family voices and the sounds of TV or planes or the cacophony of conversation or slamming doors). The baby in the womb manages incoming information from the environment by responding primitively in the earliest stages of its existence and later in a more sophisticated way. It is a delicately poised creature in relationship to its environment.

Embryologists now understand a great deal about the development of the baby's physical structure and its complex growth stages in the womb. One can marvel at this development in the remarkable photographs in Lennart Nilsson's book *A Child Is Born*. It's a wonderful book to follow during the course of pregnancy.

Three distinct stages of development are described by embryologists as the *inactive, active* and *reactive* stages. During the first *inactive stage* no movement occurs at all, but the skeletal structure and the nervous system of the tiny human embryo is developing rapidly. Then, when the skeletal muscles have become responsive to direct electrical stimulation, the organism is able to respond with movement.

At four weeks, the fetal heart begins to beat, even as it continues to elaborate. Electrical activity can be observed in the tiny brain, the first organ to develop. The digestive tract and blood circulation system are developing. By the fifth week the buds of arms and legs begin to appear and develop rapidly in the first two months. Face, eyes, nose, lips, tongue and teeth can be seen in less than an inch of human being! Tiny fingers and hands follow in the second month. Muscles begin to expand and contract. At this stage, all the elemental structures exist for further complex elaboration.

The next stage is called the active stage because there is more spontaneous activity. Slow bending of the neck and trunk is occurring in this small being. After six or seven weeks of gestation, chemicals in the brain and in other parts of the body begin to carry messages back and forth. As the tiny brain begins to function, it begins to direct movement. At seven-and-a-half weeks, the unborn baby can turn its head to the side.

During the next or reactive stage, direct sensory stimulation evokes responses in the muscular system, and reflexes of different types appear. Chamberlain speaks of it as the first sensitivity to touch. Reflexes are observable between the middle of the seventh and the beginning of the eighth weeks of gestation, when the unborn baby will respond to unpleasant sensations. It will bend its trunk and extend its arms and shoulders in order to move away. It jerks and kicks. Sensitivity in other parts of its tiny body follows.

At the base of the baby's future awareness is the brain and nervous system. All the incredible human faculties that help us make sense of the world—speech, sensory perceptions, memory, self-awareness—depend on complicated interactions within our nervous system *before* we are born, some developing quite early in our gestation.

The basis of the central nervous system and other organs such as the heart begin to form after the second week and develop rapidly. A strict time sequence is involved. Thus, any interference in the developmental process has varying effects depending on the time when the interference occurs. Effects are potentially positive or negative.

Sometime between the tenth to twelfth weeks, the unborn baby begins to move spontaneously in the womb. It uses all parts of its tiny body, rolling from side to side, extending and flexing its spine and neck, kicking its legs and waving its arms. Its vestibular system begins to form. This important part of the nervous system has to do with balance and gravity. This early development allows the baby to begin "practicing" all kinds of movement as it moves in its womb sanctuary. This movement seems to be readying a baby for postnatal activity. Muscles and motion are being tested and trained.

Between the eleventh and twelfth weeks, the baby moves its face away from a stimulus, instead of merely moving from side to side. By seventeen weeks, the unborn baby shows definite sensitivity to touch in all parts of its body. Films reveal that a fourteen-week-old reacts negatively to intrusions into its uterine environment by frowning and grimacing. Tiny as it is, it reacts.

Some prenatal researchers suggest that these spontaneous, voluntary and surprisingly graceful motions are examples of intuitive and self-expressive behavior. Touching the soft fleshy inner surface of the uterine wall, the umbilical cord, and its own body is a human being's first experience of relationship to another object. The uterus is not sensitive to touch, so the baby's kicking and poking is registered as discomfort by the mother only when the uterine wall is stretched out to the abdominal wall. Until about the twenty-eighth to thirty-second week, the unborn's movement will be free and unrestricted in its fluid world. Thereafter, the amniotic fluid begins to diminish, and its own growth makes comfort more difficult to achieve.

The unborn infant attunes to its mother's activity, and some of what we know about "behavior" in the womb is based on studies of movement patterns of the unborn baby. Swiss pediatrician Dr. Stirnimann, in his studies of the sleeping patterns of the unborn, discovered that the baby adjusted to its mother's sleeping patterns and slept when she slept and synchronized with her rhythms. He monitored a group of pregnant women with opposite sleeping patterns, those who were early-morning people and those who liked to go to bed late and rise late. The post-birth studies revealed that the early-riser mothers had babies who awoke early, and those whose mothers slept late were late sleepers, as he had suspected. It appeared that the synchronization of their rhythms was a continuation of their prebirth pattern.

At the end of the first trimester, the baby is three-and-one-half inches long, and weighs one ounce. It is active in its womb environment. It kicks, twists its feet, and even curls its newly emergent toes. Finer movement becomes possible. The baby can bend its tiny arms at the wrist and at the elbow and can make a fist with its tiny hands. Even its face is mobile, frowning, pursing its lips, opening its mouth and even squinting, despite the fact that its eyes are still sealed shut.

The baby's capacities develop rapidly, from mouth-opening at nine-and-one-half weeks to the swallowing of amniotic fluid as early as the twelfth week.

At the end of twelve weeks, the quality of response changes; it is an important age benchmark. Movements become graceful and fluid as they are in a newborn, and reactions become more vigorous. Examples of behaviors in the womb would be: grasping, sucking, swallowing, startling, turning toward a mild stimulation.

At this point, each baby's behavior differs in its womb environment as its personality emerges, since the actual structure of muscles, which follows an inherited pattern, varies from baby to baby. In all babies, however, the early simple reflexes gradually combine to yield increasingly complex "reactive" patterns until smooth, coordinated behavior develops.

The unborn baby sucks its thumbs, fingers, or toes from about fourteen weeks on, and sips the amniotic fluid in which it floats. In this period, it will begin to breathe amniotic fluid in and out of its mouth in liquid breathing. In its earliest breathing practice, some babies can be seen on the sonogram, the window to the womb, to be sucking their thumbs. In fact, some babies are such active thumbsuckers that they are born with calluses on their sucking thumb. By the eighth and ninth month, an active unborn baby will drink six to eight pints of amniotic fluid a day, receiving nourishment from its properties. An analysis of the amniotic fluid shows that it contains protein and sugar.

The sense of taste is developed early in the sequence of womb existence, although it may not exist in adult terms. At two months, taste buds begin to appear and in another month reach adult sensitivity. It is thought that they are in operation at fifteen weeks. Swallowing commences at twelve weeks. The experiences of swallowing, tasting, and sucking, therefore, exist for about six months of uterine life. The unborn even has preferences, preferring sweet tastes and rejecting sour or bitter tastes. (It is interesting to note that some tribal taboos prohibit a pregnant woman from eating anything bitter.) When a bitter substance is injected into the amniotic fluid, investigators have observed a baby to stop drinking or swallowing and to increase drinking when saccharine is introduced. A "sweet tooth" seems to be innate. At the first feeding after birth, the newborn is more practiced than anyone gives it credit for, since for several months in the womb it has known how to find its mouth with its fingers. The experience of sucking and swallowing in the womb helps the baby to nurse immediately after birth. Yet, it is not surprising that such survival behavior is practiced *in utero*.

The cerebral cortex is developed between the twenty-eighth and thirty-second week *in utero*. But the brain starts its development very early—appearing at about three weeks. The top end of the spinal cord blossoms into a brainstem—the lower portion of the brain. During the first seven weeks it grows rapidly, before a mother may know she has conceived. Midbrain and lowerbrain expand, growing out of that merge, a little above the brainstem. The cerebral cortex, the wrinkled outer surface of the forebrain, is the last evolutionary development of the human brain—the seat of thinking, feeling, remembering. It allows for the expansion of the brain to encompass the multiplication of brain cells (neurons). These various cells connect with other neighboring cells, forming communication functions. Chemical miracles occur as neurotransmitters exchange messages. Signals speed back and forth through a lacy network of nerves and arrive at the right muscles, glands, and organs in an orderly and timely way. Measurements of brain waves prove that the unborn baby's cortex is working. These show that the brain responds to stimulation of vision, touch, and hearing no later than the seventh month *in utero*. Neuroscientist Dominick Purpura, Dean of Albert Einstein Medical College in the Bronx, New York, reports that the neural circuits are as developed at this point as they will be in the newborn baby. Growth continues, of course. He believes that consciousness and awareness may be present at this point.

At the time of "quickening"—20 weeks or so—a mother-to-be will feel the flutterings of fetal activity—a most welcome sign. The baby twists and turns and kicks. A pregnant woman is quite aware of her baby's gyrations in the womb and will feel the jab of an elbow or a foot or the baby's head. She will also find her baby is responsive to pressure and touch.

At twenty-eight to thirty-two weeks, the baby's movements are fleeting, with mild avoidance responses to light and sound. There is no definite sleeping or waking pattern. At thirty-two to thirty-six weeks, there are strong responses to light and sound and definite periods of drowsy wakefulness alternating with activity. The emergence of a true sleep-waking cycle in the eighth month is considered by fetologists to be a critically important developmental transition. Babies in the womb may dream more often than adults, and just like adults during dream cycles they can be observed to smile and grimace and to be squirmy and restless. We know this from brain wave studies and REM patterns of prematurely born babies who dream almost all the time they sleep.

Do babies *in utero* see? From the sixteenth week onwards, the unborn child is sensitive to light. The womb is not completely dark; a red glow of light penetrates through the mother's body. If a bright light is shone on the mother's abdomen in line with its vision, the baby will have a startle reaction and avoid the light, and its heartbeat rate will also elevate. The light appears to be an intrusion. However, if the light is soft, the baby will turn toward it slowly and will not startle. At twenty-eight weeks patterns are perceived from pressure of the uterine fluids on the eyes. Much is being studied, however, about the newborn's ability to see immediately after birth. In his studies, Robert Frantz of Case Western University found that immediately after birth the newborn attends closely and selectively to what is going on around it. He says that it "begins acquiring knowledge about the environment at first look". But although the capacity for vision is advanced at birth, the visual part of cerebral cortex is not fully developed. Therefore, although a newborn can see at birth, it does not know what it sees. Many other researchers are studying the complexities of newborn sight and attention. Sir A. William Liley; the Auckland, New Zealand, pioneer in the field of fetal research, theorizes that the newborn's field of vision is restricted to 20/500, since that is the distance of the parameters of its uterine environment. A baby's immediate survival needs are close-range, reports Liley, that is, seeing its mother's face, which is about twelve inches from the breast, the distance it was accustomed to *in utero*. It grows acclimated to its world close at hand.

Active and sensitive, the mind of the unborn baby gains impressions of its uterine environment and also the world beyond, but not in adult terms. When researchers analyze how the external environment is affecting the unborn, it is studied in terms of increased fetal mobility or cardiac rate caused by stress of stimulation. For example, if its mother's abdominal wall is stimulated by vibration, the baby in the womb responds with increased movements. Not only sound vibrations, but a mother's fatigue level and emotions also will affect her unborn child. In a busy and frenetic world it is understandably difficult, yet very important, for a pregnant woman to spend some time in relaxation. A mother who is continuously overtired and stressed affects the environment of the womb metabolically. However, it is not the occasional and normal tension and worry of everyday life that causes serious problems. Studies demonstrate that chronic and continuous stress experienced by the mother during pregnancy causes secretion of "stress" hormones that may adversely affect the baby in the womb.

Although it was previously considered that gestation ran through a simple predetermined course of growth and development, it is now understood that child and mother influence *each other,* both biologically and emotionally.

Liley believes that the fetus is "in command of the pregnancy and is not a passive passenger." He says it is the unborn baby who determines the endocrine balance during gestation and initiates the necessary physiological changes in the mother's body to ensure a hospitable environment for its uterine existence. The baby assumes which way it will lie in the womb in response to different stimuli; it influences its own birthing time (by individual response to the levels of various hormones passing between it and its mother) and which way it will present in labor. If one observes the position a newborn chooses as it lies naked on the bed before sleep, one can see the position it preferred in the womb, says Liley.

One of the questions that remains, of course, is how the perturbations of normal life felt in the womb ultimately affect the baby developing in the womb, as well as its adult response patterns in later life. Just as the experience of a particular smell often sweeps us back to seemingly forgotten incidents and feelings, it may be that our psyches are connected to deeply etched intrauterine sensory experience, stored within our bodies, which may be evoked and may continue to unconsciously influence our behavior in subtle ways. Psychiatrist and expert on child development Dr. Daniel Stern, says it is "the self and its boundaries" that "are at the heart of philosophical speculation on human nature." All of our social experience is deeply influenced by our sense of self and its counterpart, our sense of other. Accumulating evidence points to this conclusion. But how does this knowing begin? Anthropologist and Professor Charles Laughlin questions, "Does culture actually begin to be inculcated while the child is still in the womb and does the inculcation process accelerate during the first months after birth?"

As we have seen, many new therapies are enabling people to reaccess birth memories. In the next decades, through the compilation of this information and of the memories of small children, and as more investigative studies are collated, even more answers will be found.

Therefore, many of a woman's normal habits and attitudes must be reexamined during pregnancy to ensure the psychological and physical well being of her baby as it develops in the womb. Fortunately, a pregnant woman can now benefit from a quantity of published research on the deleterious and tragic effects of radiation, drugs, alcohol, smoking and poor nutrition on the development of her baby in the womb. If its mother is a drinker, is a smoker, or uses drugs, the development of her baby will be negatively affected. These maternal habits have vital consequences.

A baby's breathing capacity in the womb is one of the earliest behaviors to be affected by its mother's lifestyle. Her cigarette habit constricts her blood vessels and reduces the amount of oxygen her baby will receive. It might even be born prematurely or underweight as a result. Investigations by Sontag's group as early as 1935 demonstrated that eight to ten minutes after a mother finishes her cigarette, the fetal heartbeat increases thirty-nine beats per minute. But, more surprising, Dr. Michael Lieberman, in a modification of the Sontag study reported in a 1970 review of prenatal development, demonstrated that even before the mother lit her cigarette and started to smoke, the baby's heartbeat increased in anticipation of the event, simply as a result of the mother being shown the cigarette and reacting to the *idea* of smoking! It is believed that the mother's heartbeat might increase in anticipation of the actual smoking of the cigarette, or that an "adrenal-like drug" crosses the placental barrier and stimulates the fetal heart. A definite response occurs. The implications of this observation of an indirect cause-and-effect fetal response are startling and far-ranging.

Many kinds of drugs present a problem in the womb. They pass through the mother's bloodstream and filter through to the unborn baby. Any adult dosage is too much for the tiny fetus *in utero*. We are discovering how damaging a mother's drug habit may be to her unborn baby. The drug passes through the placenta and affects the baby as well. The anguish of a newborn addicted to drugs, particularly crack, is profoundly painful and causes profound physiological and psychological damage.

Chemical substances in medication and drugs administered to a mother cross the placental barrier and lodge in the unborn baby's brain and body in very different proportions to a mother's larger structure. It is only recently that we have discovered to what extent the placenta is a transfer organ rather than a barrier organ. The concentration of medication required for a mother's body exceeds the concentration for the child she is carrying. Her more complex system also has the capacity to break down the drugs she has ingested and to transform them into other substances that can be absorbed into tissues in a useful form. However, a tiny being developing in the womb does not have this capability. Drugs that pass through to them are not metabolized and affect them in quite a different way. Caffeine is another example of this. French studies on the effects of caffeine on the baby indicate that the caffeine intensifies to four times its strength when transferred to the baby.

From what we know, it seems clear that during pregnancy *all* drugs should be carefully considered and not used unless absolutely necessary for a mother's health. In the normal course of our day, we take pills for so many ailments that most of us are unaware of the quantity and variety that we use. Among them are antacids, antihistamines and barbiturates. Pregnant women in the United States often take four or five different forms of medications during the nine months, eighty percent of which are over-the-counter drugs. Ill effects have been observed by obstetricians with various complications for the infant. In varying amounts, and at various times during gestation and birth, each of these has been found to have deleterious effects for a baby's development. New research continues to produce additional warnings about the dangerous effects of drugs and other lifestyle-related hazards on the mother and the baby. For example, through her lifestyle a mother may transmit the AIDS virus to her unborn child. Much less well understood, however, are the possible negative effects on human development of more subtle environmental factors, such as stress, sound, light, and pollution.

The baby hears a great deal of sound in the womb, since auditory capacities develop early. The baby is highly sensitive to sound at twenty-five weeks, and its reactions are numerous. In fact, the inner ear is completely developed by midpregnancy and the unborn baby probably begins hearing at about twenty weeks. The womb, in fact, is quite a noisy place. The amniotic fluid serves as a more effective sound conductor than air, amplifying the sounds both inside and outside the womb. There is great activity inside the mother's body. The unborn child hears and feels the rhythmic pulsations of her blood coursing through the arteries and the placenta. It hears the rhythmic pounding of her heart and of its own, which beats twice as fast as hers. And it hears the rumblings of its mother's last meal traveling through her intestines and bowels. These sounds have been discovered through recordings made inside the body. The sound of its mother's heartbeat will be the most constant vibration and rhythm an unborn baby will experience in its nine months of bounded environment, representing a basic *in utero* continuity. Imagine the reverberating sound in the watery environment transmitted to the developing baby's body. One three-year-old "remembering" womb life spoke of the sounds he heard: "moo-din, pom, pom".

A study by noted pediatrician Dr. Lee Salk in the early 60s attested to the importance of the comforting sound of the maternal heartbeat in a newborn hospital nursery. Investigators learned, as they suspected, that when a heartbeat tape was played, the newborn babies were comforted. They stopped crying and became more relaxed.

From childhood into adulthood, primal experience seems to attune our sensibilities in appreciation of musical beats and drum rhythms. Adults prefer 50 to 90 beats per minute, which is interestingly the rate of the human heartbeat. I am reminded of a workshop I led in the early 70s in a Florida mental hospital. The first morning of the group, I observed a scuffle when several group members entered the room and chose seats. Each day thereafter, one particularly disturbed patient arrived first and sat down in the seat she had won in the scuffle—a chair backed up to a window air conditioner. I assumed she enjoyed the rush of cool air at its source. On the third day, someone beat her to "her" chair. After the group meeting, I settled into the chair myself to sense what was so special about it. I was surprised to find the vibration and rhythmic beat of the motor very comforting, similar to the drumbeats of jazz drummers and ethnomusicians and, I imagined, to the sound of a human heartbeat.

A baby responds actively to a wide variety of sounds and vibrations in frequencies higher and lower than can be heard by the adult ear. A baby's movement tends to be gentled by low frequencies and excited by high frequencies. For example, when Doppler ultrasound is used to monitor the heart rate of the unborn, it is observed to increase activity. However, ultrasound used for imaging does not affect a baby's activity in the womb. Other sounds do, however, such as music.

One of the earliest signs of hearing involved the playing of music in a London maternity hospital to unborn babies between four and five months, reports audiologist Michele Clements in her 1977 studies. She said that Beethoven, Brahms and hard-rock made them restless; Vivaldi and Mozart calmed them. In his studies, Liley found that from the twenty-fifth week of gestation, the unborn will jump in rhythm to a beat.

To the baby in the womb, the many sounds it hears together may seem contrapuntal. The vibration of a washing machine, for example, can stimulate extreme activity. So will the tapping vibration of water on the sides of the bathtub as its mother bathes, or the sound of her typewriter or concert music, especially loud percussion music. As a result, the fetal heartbeat can increase by ten or more beats per second in response to the sounds and vibrations. Just imagine all the diverse sounds and vibrations a baby is exposed to in a day in its womb environment.

Bombarded by sounds in the womb, a baby may begin to select and exercise preferences about what feels comfortable to its sensibilities. Some pregnant women have reported that they were forced to leave concerts when their babies responded to the sound of percussion instruments with violent kicking. Earlier during life in the womb, loud sharp noises produced close to its mother's abdomen will startle an unborn baby, but it will move toward a soft humming noise. In tests performed by Sontag, a startle response was produced in the fetus when a sound was applied to the abdominal wall of the mother. An immediate acceleration of the baby's heart rate coincided with the sound. They concluded that the baby perceived the sound directly rather than as a reaction to the mother's reaction to the sound, because the change of endocrine products in her blood could not be so rapidly transferred to the baby.

Dr. T. Berry Brazelton, Professor of Pediatrics at Harvard, observes that when newborn, a baby exhibits strong responses to its new environment immediately after delivery. Its responses are an indication of the selective behavior it has already exercised during its uterine experience. For instance, says Brazelton, in the delivery room newborn infants may react to a loud noise once, but, on hearing it the second and third times, will tune it out. Babies will quickly temper their startle reaction and turn toward a more comfortable sound, such as a soft voice. "It is able to make distinctions that correspond to the quality of light and sound." Newborn infants have the ability to respond to sounds from the left and right but are especially accurate about sounds from straight ahead. Other researchers suspect this ability is innate.

Sounds from outside the womb, which comprise a mother's daily activity, affect the unborn also. Therefore, prenatal experience may well be affected in part by mundane things like motion picture sounds, the sound and vibrations of hours of television, vacuum cleaners, voices raised in family arguments, as well as sonic booms, roaring airplanes and the complex hubbub of a city. Not only do babies hear them directly from the source through the walls of the mother's body and react to their experience of them, but they also react to their mother's emotional and physical response to those sounds.

A fascinating study done by psychologists Anthony DeCooper and Melanie Spence at the University of North Carolina implies that an unborn baby in the later part of gestation will listen to a story and will "remember" it in some particular way. It may be an example of learning in the womb. Mothers-to-be were asked to read aloud Dr. Seuss' *The Cat In The Hat* twice a day for six weeks *before* birth. Several days after birth, the newborn babies were exposed to tapes of two Dr. Seuss' stories through earphones. One was *The Cat In The Hat,* the story their mother had read aloud, the other an unfamiliar Dr. Seuss story. Each baby was equipped with a special nipple that enabled them to switch the story they were hearing by sucking slower or more rapidly. A surprising group of ten babies out of twelve altered their sucking speed to find the familiar story. Of course, the researchers do not know precisely what was familiar—words, tone, intonation, although they feel it suggests that the babies remembered the familiar story and preferred it.

Does television have an effect on prenatal memory? One Los Angeles woman reported that her unborn child became just as involved in a TV soap opera as she was. After her baby was born she discovered that this same program had a calming effect on her baby. The baby apparently recognized the theme music and watched quietly. An Irish medical researcher, Peter Hepper of the Laboratory for Recognition Research at Queen's University in Belfast, worked with babies of loyal soap-opera watchers and observed a pattern of fetal learning behavior so repeatable that he named it "fetal 'soap' addiction." A newborn, says Hepper, clearly indicates through its behavior that it has become familiar with the first few bars of a soap opera theme while still *in utero*. The infant of a mother who watched daily is likely to stop crying when it hears the first few bars of the theme music and to focus rapt attention on the screen, while a nonwatcher's baby will continue crying.

Dr. Henry Truby, a child-language researcher, says that babies "overhear" their mother's conversations from within the womb. Truby, Professor of Pediatrics, Linguistics and Anthropology at the University of Miami, suggests that the linguistic environment of the last few months influences infant speech and language in childhood. In research done on a sabbatical leave in Sweden, Truby and his colleagues determined that the unborn baby hears during its final four and one-half months in the womb, perhaps even earlier. It is particularly sensitive to its mother's voice or the vibrations of it, since it is a daily part of its womb existence. According to Truby, cadences of the "mother tongue" heard *in utero* are carried over in the speech of children when they learn to talk. A sound-analysis instrument can detect such elements of speech when they are too subtle for the human ear to hear. For Truby, this suggests that some kind of prenatal language learning occurs.

The unborn responds to the pitch of its mother's voice. Acoustical sound prints produce "cry-prints" of the baby's sounds in the womb that are as unique as fingerprints. Indications are that the unborn baby is exercising its vocal system in preparation for life outside the womb. In the womb, a baby can more easily hear the high-pitched tone of its mother's voice than the lower register of its father's. Since sound is transmitted to the fetus more readily by bone conduction than by air conduction, a father must get close to the sound chamber of the womb environment to be heard. While sensitivity to high frequencies are developed in the womb, a child does not attune to lower frequencies until puberty.

Dr. Alfred Tomatis, a pioneering French professor of psycholinguistics, has been working with disturbed children in his clinic in Cagnes-Sur-Mer on the French Riviera. He treats young children (from one to twelve) who seem to have been traumatized by difficult pregnancies or births. In a thoughtfully designed chamber recreating the womb, these troubled children move through a "rebirthing" or "reparenting" experience. The small environment is a warm, pear- or egg-shaped environment resembling the womb. After being massaged with oil, a child is immersed in a bath of womb temperature. Colored lights are used to soothe his or her emotions. In this womb-like environment, the child listens to a recording of its mother's voice. First her voice is heard through the amniotic shield, and then it gradually becomes more familiar as it is heard by the child in its present form. Following this experience, the therapist uses a form of play and art therapy to work through the early trauma. The success rate for improvement of the children's well being is high—about 70 percent. Tomatis believes that hearing one's mother's voice in the womb environment is an important source of nurture, a kind of "vocal food", as well as basic to our future capacity to hear, speak, and even read. In 1974 William Condon and L. W. Sanders used high tech sonargraphic cameras to photograph newborns listening to their mother's speech. Their study found that a baby's movements were synchronized with its mother's speech.

These studies and many more that continue to appear indicate that patterning of infant behavior occurs before birth and that a form of learning begins in the womb that affects their lives and future development. Before birth babies respond to complex biochemical influences *and* to environmental influences such as movement, light and sound. They are delicately tuned organisms long before their transition to the outside world, with a predisposition to various responses. Learning expert Lewis Lipsitt of Brown University maintains that a newborn is "about as competent a learning organism as he can become."

"If the fetus can respond," say Mortimer G. Rosen and Lynn Rosen in their book *Your Baby's Brain before Birth*, "and, in addition, is in a state of development so that each response is more aptly called learning, then indeed the fetus—in the broadest sense of the word—is learning prior to birth. This must be said cautiously, since we do not learn *in utero* in terms of 1 + 1 = 2, or ABC. But perhaps marked environmental changes can shape later learning, ability, development and function of the fetal brain."

The possibility that the tiny being developing in the womb becomes conscious and aware, is impressionable and learning as it grows in its womb environment has profound physiological, psychological, and social implications. By becoming sensitive to its capacities, we as parents and as supportive others in a social community can create conditions that foster feelings of trust, security, and well-being in our children, even before they are born. The more we honor and nurture a baby during its sojourn in the womb, the more likely each child will be able to reach its fullest potential as it continues to develop after birth. Parents have an important role in influencing and shaping the future well-being of their child; and as a society, we need to actively support this family effort.

The Tree of Life

Lie on the floor and find a relaxed and comfortable position. Uncross your arms and legs so your energy can flow through your body. Gently close your eyes.... Take a deep breath and let it go, inhale and exhale, take another deep breath and let it go. If thoughts of your busy day intrude, allow them to drift away with an exhaled breath and bring your attention back to your breathing.... inhale and exhale, breathe gently, become aware of your breath moving in and out of your body.

Imagine your body as a vessel through which love flows. Now, imagine the roots of a large tree; follow these roots to the base of the tree and then up its trunk to its widespread branches. This is the Tree of Life, your life, with its roots deep in the earth and its branches reaching towards the sun and the moon. This tree's growth echoes the rhythms of nature, the cycles of life. You are part of that cycle, you are carrying the past forward in your seed, you are part of the endless cycle in the human family and also you are a unique part of a personal family.... Who else in your family has hair like yours? Will your baby? Who else has hands like yours? Will your baby? Choose now another family characteristic you like: will it be passed on?

Take a path that leads back in time; pick a recent time or a time long ago. Trust the image that appears for you, trust that it is all right to be there and that you are safe. Look around! Where are you? What do you see? What do you hear? What do you smell? There is a person walking toward you, you recognize this person as an ancestor of yours. Introduce yourself and your baby too. Ask about the people in your family, where they lived, the work they did, the way they played. Ask about family traditions and family dreams, and as the music carries you along, be open to discovering something new about your family....

Now thank your relative and say farewell. Slowly come back to this room: feel the floor beneath you, feel the air stirring, sense the light in the room. When you are ready, slowly open your eyes: look around the room, stretch and sit up, recall your feeling during this meditation now. Many different images and feelings may have arisen. Share them with your partner.

44

3

ONE BECOMES TWO BECOMES THREE:
WOMEN AND MEN
BECOME MOTHERS AND FATHERS

If the thought, the money, the religious enthusiasm, now expended for the regeneration of the race, were wisely directed to the generation of our descendants, to the conditions and environments of parents and children, the whole face of society might be changed before we celebrate the next centennial of our national life.

If there is a class of educators who need special education for their high and holy calling, it is those who assume the responsibility of parents. Shall we give less thought to the creation of an immortal being than the artist devotes to his statues or landscape? We wander through the galleries in the old world, and linger before the works of the great masters, transfixed with grace and beauty, the glory and the grandeur of the ideals that surround us; and with equal preparation, greater than these are possible in living, breathing humanity. The same thought and devotion in real life would soon give us a generation of saints, scholars, scientists, statesmen; of glorified humanity; such as the world has not seen. To this hour, we have left the greatest event of life to chance...

A child's first right is to be well born of parents sound in body and mind....

from *Practical Housekeeping:*
A Careful Compilation of Tried and Approved Recipes, **1881**

The period of pregnancy is a crucial time; just how is it culturally patterned? What is the effect of our society and individual psychological development on the family? How do they inter-act? How does the culture prepare parents for childbearing and parenting?

Pregnancy is a time of elation, confusion and anxiety, when profound changes are occurring in a couple's sense of them-selves, their feelings about each other and their responsibilities in the society. They need support, guidance, time, tenderness and wisdom from others more experienced than themselves. But they can't rely on their parents' wisdom as societies have done in the past. In a rapidly changing world, their parents' experience about relationships and childrearing often has become obsolete and less useful than in former periods of time. Often parents are too far away in attitude and in geography. In our polyglot, fast-moving culture, mobility, intermarriage between people of different backgrounds, changing lifestyles and values, and separation from regional and religious traditions means that a couple has no uni-fied cultural heritage to draw upon for traditional birth customs and attitudes. There seems to be no one to go to for support dur-ing this journey into the unknown as bodies change and emo-tions seesaw. In the vacuum that exists, cultural mythology seems to prevail from TV, Hollywood or magazines—a confusing mix-ture. A couple's bewilderment in trying to have a balanced per-sonal experience amidst the wash of these confusing messages that may not tally with their own experience raises the normal anxiety level that accompanies pregnancy and birth.

In her pregnant state, as a woman becomes a mother, she may have many conflicting feelings and thoughts, and it is likely they will be positive, negative and ambivalent messages, such as the following:

- I feel so sexy, does everybody know?
- I *want* to be this way forever: peaceful, serene.
- I'm an integral part of the universe. It's hard to explain.
- I want a lot of cuddling. I feel like a kitten who wants to be stroked.
- It's the first time I've had a purpose in my life. I feel privi-leged to be carrying and nourishing a new life.

- Even when *I'm* not doing anything, my body is making a new person!

- I want to feel like a goddess, be waited on, be the center of attention.

- This baby will make such a difference in my life and my relationship.

- I've been waiting to become a mother my whole life.

- The whole meaning of my life has changed; things will never be the same.

- I love being pregnant.

- I don't really like the bother of being pregnant, I'd just like to have the baby here now.

- How will I know what to do?

- I'm afraid I will be this way forever: needy, dependent, emotional, anxious.

- I'm afraid of the responsibility of the child.

- I'll be fat and ugly forever.

- He won't love me anymore; he'll find someone else to love.

- Having a baby will wreck my career.

- I don't know who I am any more.

- I feel as if I'm moving into the unknown; it's scary.

- I feel slow and stupid.

- We'll never have any time together after the baby is born.

- I'm afraid I'm going to die.

* * * *

During this period of gestation, while the baby in the womb is making its remarkable journey into becoming, a mother is also undergoing an extraordinary process directly related to a new being growing within her. We tend to focus on the actual birth because it is dramatic and because we can see it happening and others are involved in it culturally. But—just as for the baby the birth event may be considered a link between two states of consciousness (womblife and autonomy)—for the mother, too, it is also a bridge between two states of consciousness (pregnancy and parenthood). She senses she is part not only of family history, but of the grand forces of nature, of evolution.

A body of knowledge is accumulating that helps us map the complex dimensions of her naturally altered state of consciousness during the childbearing year. We are becoming increasingly aware that pregnancy and birth can precipitate transcendent, ecstatic emotional states, similar to those caused by other intense experiences such as orgasm or the creation of art, contact with nature, or a spiritual experience. She may transcend the ordinary, familiar sense of self, to achieve an extraordinary understanding of being one with the cosmos.

Women sense their autonomy; at the same time they experience being part of all that is, ever has been, ever will be. These experiences move beyond ordinary time and space. Ego boundaries dissolve. These are the states we read about in mystical literature. We find they are accessible to each of us. The expansion and deepening of personal awareness is one of the unexpected and remarkable aspects of the birth process. Psychologist Abraham Maslow called these sensations "peak experiences." We invite these states all too rarely, and therefore their manifestation can be unfamiliar and frightening at first, as well as ecstatic.

Knowledge of the emotional stages that an expectant mother will pass through during the year may help her to realize the peak aspects of the experience of pregnancy and birth, even as she confronts troubling ones. For the father too, important psycho-spiritual and even bodily changes occur.

For the pregnant woman, doubts about whether she ought to have a child at all makes her situation even more difficult. In her mother's generation, motherhood was unquestioningly desirable and esteemed. But today a pregnant woman probably deals with the need to work and earn money, with social concerns about overpopulation and with a personal need to find her own identity and self-expression before she gets swallowed up by motherhood and domesticity. Sharing in consciousness-raising groups of the past decades has exposed the complexities of those feelings.

Until recently, perhaps only a generation ago, there were clearly delineated responsibilities and duties for men and women. In the family, men were the providers, women, the homemakers and mothers. For the last decades, however, women's expectations and cultural attitudes have changed. It is not only in two-career families that men are expected to share more responsibility for household chores, child care, and nurturing. Gone, by and large, are the close-knit two-generation families with grandparents and aunts and uncles to help. Couples have to depend on each other to handle the day's needs.

With men more involved in the "domestic" world even as they work outside the home, their feelings and emotions begin to become more visible to their partners. And they, like their partners, need nurturing, support, and extra doses of understanding. There is often greater confusion about accepting role models from past generations and more experimentation in ways of thinking about pregnancy and parenthood. Many people are finding their own answers. Hopefully, it will be a path of the heart.

* * * *

Pregnancy is a process of becoming—not only for the baby but for the mother as well. We have learned that a woman will move through predictable stages of development during pregnancy, not only biologically, but psychologically and spiritually as well. The interrelationship of these stages is becoming increasingly clear. Yet, each person goes through pregnancy in her own unique way, feeling some or most of the feelings others may feel. There may be different content in what is experienced, or the timing of what is felt may be individual. In the section that follows, I have summarized some of the most dramatic changes as they are now understood. Individual women may experience some of the following feelings. Also, each trimester has positive, negative and ambivalent feelings.

EMOTIONS AND FEELINGS DURING PREGNANCY

First Trimester (first through twelfth week)

- Ambivalence, doubts, uncertainty even when pregnancy is planned

- Joy, pride in fertility, euphoria, disbelief.

- Thoughts of abortion

- Fear of incompetence, fear of harming the developing fetus

- Bizarre food cravings

- Acceptance of pregnancy; initial rejection of pregnancy

- Vulnerability, fear of change, disruption

- Loss of control; natural process is taking over

- Increased appetite; decreased appetite, nausea, loss of weight

- Fear of dependence; concerns about trust, fear of changes in marriage relationships, fear of sexual infidelity

- Freedom in sex; heightened sexuality, (occasional fear of harming fetus during sex); disinterest in sex—too sick, too tired

- Moodiness; unpredictability; increased awe in relation to the pregnant state, emotional sensitivity, fear of miscarriage

- Increased need for love and affection

- Physical fatigue, increased need for sleep

Second Trimester (thirteenth through twenty-fourth week)

- Increased dream and fantasy activity; uncensored emotional reactions

- Heightened sexual desire

- Introspection, thoughts about the meaning of life

- Concerns about relationship with doctor and hospital

- Fascination with development of pregnancy

- Heightened awareness of unconscious processes

- Sense of excitement and reality in feeling baby's movements; awareness of irreversibility of events

- Free-floating anxiety

- Concern about balancing motherhood and career

- Thoughts about her own mother; transition from daughter to mother, with accompanying conflicts and fears

- Shift in dependency from her mother to her husband

Third Trimester (twenty-fourth through fortieth week)

- Emotions close to the surface

- Ambivalence toward changing body

- Pride in full-blown pregnancy; reveling in role of lifegiver (identification with divine aspects of motherhood, female goddess myths)

- Impatience with physical discomfort

- Need for affection and recognition of special state

- Fear of death; fear of letting go; fears about labor and delivery

- Fears of separation from the baby

- Need for security; resentment of dependency, awareness of one's own needs

- Fears of infidelity

- Fatigue

- Fear of incompetence as mother and wife

- Fear of abnormality of baby

- Anxiety about money, lifestyle, the future; preoccupation with pregnant self and developing baby

- Discomfort with increased fetal activity and size; sense of being invaded

- Insomnia; dreaming

- Awkwardness

- Reality of baby's existence; acceptance

- Nesting: excited preparation for baby's arrival, naming, fixing crib

- Start of childbirth classes

Postpartum (Reintegration)

- Need for family bonding, mother-child bonding

- Need for affection, reassurance, praise, security

- Celebratory period

- Emotional swings due to worries about competence in breast feeding, about mothering the baby, role as lover and partner

- New sense of identity needing personal integration

- Need for social reintegration with community and career

- If there are siblings, fear that there won't be enough time or love to go around

- Concern about sibling rivalry

Mothers to be may be easily confused by these positive, negative and ambivalent feelings.

It is clear that the increased hormone level during pregnancy profoundly affects a woman's body as it makes a baby. Although a pregnant woman naturally anticipates and does not wish to resist these hormonally mediated physical changes, it is the out-of-control effect of these hormones on her emotional state that she may be totally unprepared for and frightened by. She has to attune to a new rhythm as this new being within invades her body. She has to change her eating habits; she is eating for two. She has to yield to her fatigue. She has to listen to ever-changing and intensified emotional voices. In trying to maintain her equilibrium, she may resist the impetus toward the accompanying psychological changes that are preparing her for the totally new role as mother. In addition, hormonal changes that create an altered state—often a transcendent one—may be even more unfamiliar and difficult to allow. However, instead of perceiving her feelings, dreams and fantasies as aberrant or "crazy," she can be encouraged to view this period as a positive source of new understanding of herself and her world. Consciously letting go— surrendering—moving into the unknown, opening herself to the wide-ranging new experiences and changes move her through an important personal transformation.

The expectant mother is undeniably undergoing a normal crisis of transition. Everything in her life is changing. This crisis has a dual nature, representing both danger and opportunity. "Crisis," says Richard Grossman in *Choosing and Changing,* "can only be avoided by those who refuse to undertake the journey of becoming." It is a time of questioning, of reexamining one's life and the meaning of existence.

One pattern frightening to women during pregnancy is often a regressive return to earlier attitudes and modes of behavior. Even a woman who is mature and confident and wants a child may find herself on an emotional seesaw, swinging from positive to negative feelings toward her pregnant state and her life in general. For example, she may normally accept the necessity of her partner's business trips, but during pregnancy she may have a hard time with his absence, which may bring to exaggerated childlike feelings of insecurity and abandonment. These irrational feelings and shifts may confuse and irritate her partner, who may be beset by his own anxieties about the impending financial and emotional responsibility of parenthood.

A pregnant woman may feel unpredictably wide fluctuations of mood, resulting in outbursts of laughter, unexplained anxiety, sudden tears, depression, fearful dreams, embarrassing vulnerability or the tendency to be superstitious. Both she and her partner may find this unfamiliar behavior disconcerting, to say the least. Yet all of this behavior is normal.

Dreams and fantasies are the psyche's way to prepare a pregnant woman for the dramatic changes in the course of pregnancy. Dr. T. Berry Brazelton of Harvard University and Boston Children's Hospital and the National Commission on Children, a noted pediatrician and eminent researcher of family life, feels that the emotional anxiety and disruption of old concepts through dreams enable a pregnant woman to get ready for her new role. Increased hormonal flow intensifies her responses and opens her to significant changes in her life.

Although many of her fears may involve projections into an unknown future, others are firmly based on the changes that are taking place in her daily life. For example, she may worry about sexual attractiveness as her body swells, or about her changing relationship to her partner as they become a family, and about her imminent loss of independence as the caretaker of a tiny baby. The dependent aspects of pregnancy are already giving her intimations of this. Some parental anxiety centers, too, around the increased economic responsibility that is an integral part of parenthood. These threads converge and weave together, adding to the sum of each partner's individual anxieties. Taken one by one or all together, these questions will disturb the normal rhythms of a couple's life.

It becomes necessary to seek new ways of achieving balance and harmony and it will be necessary to confront the anxiety produced. A father-to-be may need to rearrange his schedule, as much as is feasible, in response to his partner's vulnerability at this time, a woman may need to reassure her partner that the baby is not pushing him aside. Reassurances to unspoken questions can be crucial for maintaining this important bond during a time when the self-image of each partner is threatened. Open communication, heightened sensitivity, and support are the keys.

It is not unusual for a woman to feel ambivalent in the early months as she becomes aware of the awesome and irreversible responsibility that she is undertaking. Poet Judith Thurman writes:

> I am appalled by the definiteness of motherhood. Once you
> have a child you are never, afterward, not a mother. It is as
> if you were the ocean and the child a continent that rises
> up in you—usurping your energy, attracting settlers and
> institutions, forcing you to become part of history.

Once having decided to become a parent, pregnancy is a "point
of no return."

Ambivalence is one of the most important issues to deal with
in the early (and even during the later) stages of pregnancy. The
doubts about her capacity to be a good mother, to be responsible for her child, to put her career on hold are central to early
pregnancy. Feelings of ambivalence are normal and typical.

If a woman has had a career, she is likely to feel even more
ambivalent about motherhood. She doesn't want to be cast into
the backwater that she observes young mothers existing in. She
needs to continue to develop as a whole person; she wants the
continued respect she has already earned in her field; she wants
the stimulation of a mixed community in her daily life. She
struggles with the fear that having a child will cut her off from
the "important world."

These reservations, of course, are set against powerful forces
in support of the role she is now entering. Parents, the institutions that surround her, and the media are out there on the
"motherhood bandwagon," suggesting that living out her repro-
ductive role is her only way of fulfilling herself as a woman-person. Her own psychobiology collides with societal attitudes to
reinforce that notion. These leave her little room to bring out
and examine her fears and doubts.

> Society puts a lot of pressure on us to have babies, and
> smiles approvingly when we become pregnant....[If] we
> have negative feelings about being mothers...we tend to
> deny ourselves our legitimate anxieties; then sometimes
> they appear after our child is born in forms we're not
> prepared to handle.

Confronting these ambivalent feelings is central to the child's
future well-being. Research studies show that "an unwanted

child" is a far more serious problem and that the child may be impaired psychologically, emotionally, even chemically. It is wise to seek psychological counselling if the mother's or father's feelings are intense.

In Grete L. Bibring's ten-year studies of the psychological aspects of pregnancy, at Beth Israel Hospital in Boston, it was discovered that *all* women exhibited significant and far-reaching psychological changes when pregnant. It is apparent from the work of Bibring, Therese Benedict, Sheila Kitzinger, Niles Newton, and more recently English psychoanalyst Joan Raphael-Leff and other researchers, that there is a distinct pattern of *pregnancy consciousness*. Some women are thrown off balance more than others. And each woman's pregnancy is quite different from her previous one, not only because she herself has changed physiologically, but also because her social and psychological self-awareness is altered each time. Each baby also has different genes. Experienced nurses and midwives observe that mothers who seem to have it together during pregnancy frequently fly apart in the postpartum stage, often soon after birth. These health professionals feel that confronting emotions during pregnancy is crucial to the adjustment into parenthood. It is interesting to note that pregnant women who are referred to psychotherapists for help during the course of pregnancy appear to achieve striking therapeutic results. Therapists report that problems are close to the surface during this open and receptive time and can be handled in relatively few sessions. It is as if she is more able to confront her "shadow side." Although the content of such therapy may be similar to that presented by severely neurotic patients, who might more to confront the same material, it is handled far more directly and easily by pregnant women. Says Dr. Gerald Caplan of Harvard's School of Community Health:

> All kinds of fantasies and needs and wishes, which were previously unconscious, are now allowed out into consciousness, without producing as much anxiety as you would expect. It is as though during this period, the ego,

probably as a result of its increased strength due to metabolic changes, does not mind living with these previously unconscious appetites.

—"Concepts of Mental Health"

A crucial psychological theme during pregnancy is a woman's relationship to her own mother. The intimate dependency of her infancy and childhood has evolved into a more independent relationship during the course of her puberty, adolescence and young womanhood. At this point, the mother-daughter relationship reaches a plateau. Although both the positive and negative aspects of the old relationship may remain, the mother and daughter may be more distant—both emotionally and geographically. During pregnancy, a woman may long to resume the old dependent relationship with her family, particularly with her mother or a close female friend. Although she may not act on her feelings, the longing may be intense. Negative feelings may emerge also. The long-forgotten or suppressed feelings of love-hate based on early dependency reemerge during pregnancy to be faced once again. It is part of the reevaluation process of this transition. In her normal, introverted state around the time of quickening, the time when the baby's movements are felt—the first kick—her thoughts return to old unresolved feelings about her own mother. She may feel more loving or more rebellious or angrier about the frustrating relationship she has with her mother or may experience all these feelings simultaneously. She can progress in her own evolution by confronting these feelings head on, assisted by the powerful dynamics of her own biochemistry. Pregnancy becomes an opportunity to move through the dependent stage to one in which she sees herself as coequal with her mother. As the daughter, she can begin to see herself as a separate and distinct person and a potentially capable mother in her own right, entering the responsible realm of adulthood. This realization can bring her closer to accepting her mother as a distinct person as well.

Working through the unresolved feelings with her mother or on her own can allow the bond between them to develop into mutual appreciation and love and interdependency. Not everyone is fortunate in having the opportunities to work through these difficulties with their parents.

Clearing obstructed feelings with her own mother allows her to come to her own child with an openness and clarity, a clean slate, and to generously give the love that is the source of her baby's emotional health. Receiving unconditional love is the beginning of a life of trust, security and altruism for a new being coming into life,a template for later experience.

Before the birth, in essence, the expectant mother belongs to her family of origin; after the birth, she establishes her own family. She begins to weave together the threads of family origin, heritage, with the establishment of her own order.

In many other cultures, proscribed behavior helps guide parents-to-be through the transition. However, psychotherapist and transcultural psychologist Anne Hubbell Maiden, who is developing an important cross-cultural study called *Continuity of Care: Seven Stages of Birthwork,* says, "It is rare to find a culture which reports a balanced awareness of preconception, conception, gestation, birthing, bonding, infancy and early childhood, yet each has its part to offer to human well-being."

One of the cultural patterns she describes was related to her by Basque anthropologist Angeles Arrien. It offers integrated and positive rituals. The Basque people of Spain treasure birth and their customs honor it as "a sacred art." Traditionally, Basque couples wait until they are in their 30s or 40s to have their families, feeling they are more mature (as do many American couples today). During the pregnancy, the parents-to-be attune to their baby in the womb and begin to tell each other stories aloud about the baby and its life so that the baby can hear. They also sing songs that will be repeated during the birth and will be sung to the baby after the birth. The father stays in close touch with his unborn child during the pregnancy and may identify so closely with his partner that he experiences some manifestations of pregnancy.

The entire extended family gathers at the birth, including siblings, aunts, uncles, grandparents. All are considered birth attendants. The environment is carefully considered and when weather permits, the birth takes place out of doors, often near a running stream. In fact, they have very complex ideas about rites of passage in relation to the environment. Concentric circles are formed around the mother and father and siblings. There is a merry accompaniment of music: singing, chanting, drums and flutes, plus storytelling and jokes to cheer the laboring mother. They speak of massaging the mother and baby with laughter. All the family stay together for seven days—and at the end of the ritual week celebrate with the entire village.

In other cultures, traditional patterns of behavior acknowledge a need for the familiarity, wisdom and support of one's own mother. For example, in the Punjab in India and in Botswana, a pregnant woman leaves her husband and her mother-in-law, with whom she may still feel shy, and travels to the home of her birth to be with her own mother and the village midwife, whom she has known throughout her life. In the United States, contemporary women are no less in need of traditional guidance, expertise and love and emotional support to alleviate their fears of this unknown and unpredictable period.

The question "Who am I?" arises quite normally during this period.

- Who am I in relation to my changing body and the being growing inside me?

- How can I be sure that my body will transform the invisible seed into a fetus and then into a real baby? Can I do it?

Her identity is threatened as another being grows inside her body—two people inhabiting the same body. Everything she eats, feels, even thinks is shared by her preborn baby. "Clearly," says British psychoanalyst/researcher Joan Raphael-Leff, "one of them must go." Her most primitive, unspeakable fear is that during birth the wrong one will be expelled.

- What if I am carrying a boy?

- Is it an assault on my femininity?

- Am I being possessed from within by my mate?

Some of her anxiety centers around the well-being of each member of the family. For example, if her husband is late, she may become obsessed with fear that a serious accident or unknown danger has befallen her partner. Or she may be anxious about injury to herself, may even fantasize about her own death, or that her father's flu may cause his death, or she may fear the baby will be abnormal, deformed. One member of my group reported:

> I have dreadful images of holding a deformed baby—no arms or legs—just a trunk and a beautiful face. I want to do away with it. I keep wondering if there were members of my family that were deformed and nobody ever told me.

She may fear that the baby will die during delivery or be still-born, or that the fetus will continue growing bigger and bigger inside her, until her body bursts its seams as it explodes out. These concerns progress in galloping fashion, often activated by reading a newspaper account of a disaster or watching TV news or hearing something from a friend. These frightening images come and go and then pass.

The normal anxieties of pregnancy are further aggravated by cultural messages absorbed in childhood that are hard to shake. The disparagement of women's feelings and intuition and the depreciation of women's abilities and contributions is part of the cultural climate in which we were raised. After years of being recipient of these negative attitudes, it is not surprising that many women come to childbearing with little confidence or joy.

Think about what each of us was told about our bodies and its biological/physical changes. For women, certainly family attitudes and cultural messages shape the way we feel about menstruation, intercourse and childbearing.

A patriarchal society tends to mystify what is happening because mystification keeps women uninformed and passive at a time when they most need to know what to expect and what to do. "Why such mystification?" asks the Boston Women's Health Collective. "Women, who menstruate bloodily, carry children in their wombs as animals do, give birth without obvious effort and some discomfort, are close to nature." A male-dominated culture seems threatened by the raw physicality and creates more senti-mental myths about women's sexuality, which women come to believe.

Certainly women's images of themselves in this culture have been defined for them largely by men. Men who are biologists, anthropologists, priests, and historians have described how women feel and are. But this often doesn't tally with a woman's own reality and may leave her with great doubts about herself.

For generations, women have been raised with tales of the risks of childbirth—long, difficult and painful labors, maternal death, strange infant abnormalities and birth injuries. Of course, there can be complications but it is important to remember that ninety-five percent of all births are normal. Therefore, these fears are often irrational and even subconscious. However, some are realistic, fueled by the experiences of friends. Some fears are based on contemporary obstetrical practice and inappropriate, scientifically oriented, mechanized hospital procedures—the medicalization of childbirth. Deaths and injuries however are quite rare.

Some fears are primitive, even primordial—arising from the deeper recesses of the psyche, and difficult to explain in a con-temporary context. Periodically, during pregnancy, some women may feel that their happiness arouses the envy of the gods and spirits, recalling from childhood the myths and fairy tales of supernatural beings who inflict harm on mothers and their chil-dren: the malevolent, wicked witch in "Rapunzel" in Grimm's *Fairy Tales,* who lures the baby away. Women are in touch with the shadow side of existence, as eminent Swiss psychologist Carl Jung describes it. Today, as in times past, inconsistent as it may be with our rational training, superstitious relatives and friends with roots in Central-European or Middle Eastern cultures may warn the pregnant mother that the "evil eye" will bring trouble. Psychoanalyst Helene Deutsch speaks of these primitive fears in *The Psychology of Women,* suggesting that for educated women of our civilization, to adopt superstitions seems irrational. Pregnant women nevertheless feel anxious about their fantasies of monsters and unnatural births. Despite the balance of rationality they may have previously experienced, they develop fear of magic forces and may engage in superstitious beliefs.

A mother-to-be may fear she will die in childbirth and that the baby will retain her body. Fears of death and dying fascinate and obsess many pregnant women. "I keep dreaming about my death with my monster fetus standing over me. It's horrible." Dreams of death occur often. In fact, pregnant women dream about death more frequently than their nonpregnant friends—forty percent as compared to ten percent. These dreams are dreams of transformation, death-rebirth dreams as well as dreams activated by literal fear of death. "In mythology," says Joseph Campbell, "the god of death is also the god of regeneration." That which dies is reborn. Birth and death, therefore, appear inextricably connected.

Many suggest that our fear of death begins during our profound experience of birth. Each generation gives way to the next. "There is a deep psychological association of begetting and dying," says Campbell in *The Power of Myth*. It is rooted deep in the psyche and therefore, not surprisingly, is felt by a pregnant couple. Death to one level of existence, rebirth on another plane. Death to the girl/woman, birth of the mother/woman.

In the last phase of pregnancy, typical dreams and fantasies may concern losing the baby or having it delivered in a bizarre way. These dreams and fantasies can be quite frightening. They can also be illuminating when understood in the symbolic language of dreams. Some women dream that they destroy their child or throw their baby out the window: "I had a dream that after I had my baby, I forgot all about it. I didn't feed it for days—it started to get smaller and died."

Or women may be concerned with how the baby will get out: "How is a person twenty-one inches long going to get out of me?" When she has only produced vomit, spit, urine, feces, blood from inside her body, she wonders how can she produce a good viable person, says anthropologist Joan Raphael-Leff.

The anxieties and fears take many forms during different trimesters. Early in pregnancy, a woman may be afraid that she will lose the baby; later on, she may fear that her partner will abandon her or die, leaving her alone and helpless. Intimately as she is involved with the creation of new life, it is not surprising that she is also poignantly aware of its ending.

Not only is a pregnant women close to her own unconscious process, but she appears to be connected to the deepest levels of the collective unconscious. Fantasies and dreams undoubtedly serve to guide her through the profound psychological and transpersonal changes that this passage in the life cycle involves. Her psyche and biochemistry interweave in mysterious and wondrous ways. If the concern and fascination with death is seen as an expanded awareness of continuing transition—that is, death/rebirth—then awesome fantasies, phobias and fears during pregnancy can be explored and understood in quite a different dimension. They present one with an opportunity for deeper insight into one's own life process, instead of as a crisis to be feared.

Childbearing is a heroine's journey, says Campbell, "And where we had thought to be alone, we will be with all the world." Bearing a life within one's body and giving birth is certainly a heroic deed involving the surrender of oneself to the life of another. When a woman returns from the heroine's journey, she has created a new life—a gift to give to the world. Giving yourself over to a higher principle, says Campbell, is difficult—the ultimate trial—a heroic transformation. It is what myths deal with—a transformation of consciousness—all of what you thought previously changes.

A pregnant woman questions who she is in relation to her mother who brought her into life. The transition into motherhood puts a woman in touch with the of bearing life and in turn with the mythic mother principle that gives life to forms—the creative, the nurturing, the collaborative. She identifies with mythological mother figures: earth goddesses and the Universal, or Divine, Mother.

Most subtle of all is the sense that one's psychic self is dying—the old self giving way to the new parent self—death-rebirth. Both men and women share these fears and opportunities for profound change. It is partly the subconscious process of surrendering the old self, rather than a morbid obsession with dying, that activates symbols of death and subsequent rebirth in dreams and waking consciousness. These symbolic dreams may allow her to reach beyond her unique personal experience in order to touch mystical levels of a wider human experience, enabling her to dissolve the ego boundaries which separate her from others.

It is this transpersonal aspect of childbearing that is so little discussed. Grof speaks of it. Psychologist Rollo May discusses the sense of oneness and the fears that surround intimacy in *Love and Will*, as he speaks of orgasm

> as a psychophysical symbol of the capacity to abandon one's self, to give up present security in favor of the leap towards the deeper experience—the known for the unknown. It is not by accident that the orgasm often appears symbolically as death and rebirth.

In orgasm, a deep union with our polar opposite, there is surrender. If only for seconds, one experiences the absence of ego boundaries, the transcendence of self. In Bali, in fact, the act of making love is called "becoming one." By virtue of sexual union, in the act of love, each time, we are renewed. We *are* changed. But it is frightening. As May has written:

> When we love, we give up the center of ourselves. We are thrown from our previous state into a void; and though we hope to attain a new world, a new existence, we can never be sure....We give, and give up our own center; how shall we know that we will get it back?

During pregnancy, a woman literally and symbolically has these longings and fears. The symbiosis with the baby is an experience of union for her and is reminiscent of her own gestation period in the womb. As May points out, this earliest period of union is repeated in adult life in sexual union:

> The sexual act is the most powerful enactment of relatedness imaginable, for it is the drama of approach and entrance and full union, then partial separation...then a complete reunion again. It cannot be an accident of nature

that in sex we enact the sacrament of intimacy and with-
drawal, union and distance, separating ourselves and giving
in full union again.

It is *not* an accident; it is the reiteration of an earlier relationship each of us had with our mothers. Deeply ingrained in our
memory is this archetypal theme, from which myths and fairy
tales derive. It is the template for a later union with a loved one
and with a universal presence, God, if you will.

As in the balance of opposites, on the other side of ecstasy in
love is awareness of death, and just as in ecstatic lovemaking
between a man and a woman, so too in the midst of the pleasure of the symbiotic ecstasy of mother-love, pregnant women
often fear that merging with the baby may destroy the self.

Confronting these deep arcane levels of the psyche allows a
woman to experience the primordial process of change as she
moves from merely being the child to her mother to becoming
the mother to her child as well. Death and rebirth. Allowing the
old self to die and a new self to be reborn to a new level in the
unfolding spiral of her life—as a mother.

Perhaps it is the gathering intensity of mother-love that read-
ies a woman for bonding and that also at the same time evokes
a fear of symbolic death in the immediate separation. She realizes that the baby she has nurtured and cradled within her body
for nine long months must now be surrendered. There is anxiety
connected with these feelings of separation, even though she
may feel ready for the pregnancy to be over and may know that
in losing the "fetus," she is gaining a child.

There may even be the poignant sense that as she loses the
baby within her, the child is also losing her. The relationship
must change. The harmony between mother and child is broken;
the nine-month symbiosis is over; each one of them must adjust
to their new state. A Jungian analyst describes the following
dreams reported by a pregnant patient two weeks before her
baby was born. In the first, she was in heaven and had to practice a gliding motion in order to return to earth. Though she
knew landing on earth meant death, she was forced to let go.
She landed, died and then awoke. Later, she had another dream

in which she was moving up and down on the waves of the ocean and was commanded to surrender to the movement of the waves. This dream prepared her psychologically for later surrender during childbirth.

Changing sexual needs and feelings are another major concern for a woman and her partner during the childbearing year. Feelings about ourselves as sexual beings obviously cannot be separated from the sum total of our feelings and needs and attitudes, but during pregnancy a woman may experience new and unfamiliar intensities of sexual rhythms. These hormonally stimulated changes may seem random and frightening, causing her to feel that her sexual identity is wildly fluctuating and unpredictable. Her sexual self-image may be threatened as a result. Her feelings may range from a dismaying lack of interest in sex to bewildering, all-consuming erotic feelings. It is not unusual for a woman in this state to walk down the street imagining that everyone knows how sexy she's feeling.

In general, during the first pregnancy, studies show a decrease in interest and sexual performance in the first trimester, but an increase in erotic feeling in the second trimester. In fact, eighty percent of the women questioned in a Masters and Johnson study reported greater sexual satisfaction in the second trimester, compared both to the earlier months of pregnancy, and to their experience before pregnancy. In general, many women's sexual desire decreases as pregnancy moves along as they become less comfortable. However, this varies among individuals.

Not often pointed out is that many of the physiological changes that normally occur during sexual arousal when a woman is not pregnant—such as increased blood supply in the genital region, increased vaginal lubrication, tension and erection of breasts and nipples, tilting of the uterus—are normal phenomena of the pregnant state. Thus, it may be, as Libby Colman and Elisabeth Bing suggest in their book, *Sex During Pregnancy,* that pregnant women may feel more or less "turned on" all the time. In addition pleasure may be enhanced when lovemaking is no longer affected by the need for contraception. These unusually intense and unfamiliar feelings of constant arousal may also be a source of anxiety to a woman and her partner, especially in our culture; desire for frequent sex may be interpreted as excessively demanding or "needy" behavior.

At the beginning of pregnancy, the lack of interest in sex may stem from morning sickness, fears of miscarriage, or just plain fatigue. If sex is the main form of physical expression of love and caring between partners, a woman may feel deprived of the physical touching she needs during this vulnerable time. Fondling, caressing, massaging each other are other ways to express loving and sexual feelings. It is crucial to begin to explore alternative ways to give pleasure to each other and to keep communication open. Recent books on sexuality can help a couple express and fulfill their individual needs. A man's awareness of his pregnant partner's increased needs for tenderness, affection and care can significantly reduce tensions and avoid a retreat into resentful distance, and her sensitivity to his needs are crucial as well. What affects the mother affects the baby and, just as importantly, may influence the future relationship between mother and child, father and child. Psychologist Dr. Gerald Caplan of Harvard stresses:

> We all know that a woman needs increased vitamins and proteins during pregnancy, and that if she doesn't get these she is likely to have all kinds of difficulties and complications. In just the same way, she needs increased supplies of love and affection and if she does not get them, she may have difficulty in giving love and affection to her child.

Affection, cuddling and lovemaking, if viewed in this light, are ways to nurture everyone involved; mother, father and child. It is, also, as the Yurok Indians believe, a way to teach love and tenderness in the womb. Rather than being seen as an increased demand on the expectant father, it gives him an essential, nurturing role.

Near the end of the pregnancy, most women feel needy and dependent, as do many men. Women are apt to be self-involved, introspective, consumed with the complexity of what is happening inside their bodies. Some are anxious. Many are just plain uncomfortable. Nine months may feel like a long time. Fortunately, it is not as long as the gestation period of horses or whales, 12 months, or elephants, 20-22 months.

A woman's lack of interest in sex, coupled with her increased irritability, may strain her partner's empathy to its limits. The absence of a tender way to release tension, the anxiety created by the imminence of birth, can build up to a potentially explosive situation. It is essential to be able to talk openly about what's happening. A couple's reluctance or inability to confront the anxieties and discuss the problem does not deny its importance. Honest exchange about the most intimate of human encounters is an art in which few of us are skilled. It's scary; so much seems at stake. Doctors may not be able to provide the needed solutions and it may be wise to talk to close friends, in addition to reading how others have successfully developed new ways of relating. Pregnancy support groups can be very helpful and often the best avenue for help. Those who are involved with the same problem often offer the most considered help.

How a woman or man responds to the changes of pregnancy will vary according to individual sexual appetite, family attitudes carried along from childhood, the impact of cultural myths, taboos and superstitions, and importantly, the support she receives. It is surprising to see how pervasive and influential these myths and taboos can be. They seem to be almost as pervasive in some parts of contemporary culture as they have been in isolated preliterate cultures. Sociologist Lucille Newman reports some of the prevalent beliefs she gathered in a study of pregnant women in Northern California in the late 1970's. In answer to the question, "What have you heard about prenatal influence or about how a mother's behavior can affect her unborn child?" the answers in different ethnic groups were similar even though the language and socio-economic status changed from one group to another. Interestingly, African Americans tended to validate their answers by citing personal testimony and whites by invoking a medical authority. These were some of the superstitions and taboos expressed:

- Eating strawberries will leave a strawberry mark on the child.

- If you don't get what you crave, the baby will be allergic to it.

- Smoking will make you lose the baby.

- Stay in the house during an eclipse.

- If you are frightened by a snake, your baby will look like a snake.

- If you go to a funeral, it will hurt the baby.

- Watching horror movies will affect the baby mentally.

- If you eat certain foods the baby will be insane.

- Don't cross your legs; it will make the baby blind.

According to midwife Elizabeth Gilmore, among some of the Hispanic women in Northern New Mexico:

- If you have a lot of heartburn your baby will have lots of hair.

- If you raise your arms above your head, you will cause the umbilical cord to tangle.

During pregnancy, when each partner's self-image is undergoing a change from person to the role of "parent," both partners need extra reassurance. She needs to know she is still attractive to him; he needs to know he is not being replaced by the person in the womb. A woman's view of herself and the transformation she is undergoing, of which her body is a visible manifestation, form part of the psychological climate of the baby's experience in the womb and during birth. Far from being supported and affirmed as she moves from adolescence to womanhood to motherhood, and later to menopause, a woman often has to struggle to learn about herself, about what's happening biologically, as if the workings of her body are an unmentionable, mysterious secret best concealed. Advances in the field of women's health, as a result of the women's movement, fortunately are making available to all women information about their psychology and biology. The expanding awareness will help them make intelligent and heartfelt decisions during pregnancy and about the way they want to give birth.

A woman's sense of herself as a sexual person is delicate and constantly shifts throughout her life, in ways that men do not experience so acutely. A quotation by an Abyssinian woman recorded by the anthropologist Leo Frobenius in the early twentieth century illustrates this idea:

> How can a man know what a woman's life is? A woman's life is quite different from a man's. God has ordered it so. A man is the same from the time of his circumcision to the time of his withering. He is the same before he has sought out a woman for the first time, and afterwards. But the day a woman enjoys her first love cuts her in two. She becomes another woman on that day. The man is the same after his first love as he was before. The man spends a night by a woman and goes away. His life and body are always the same. The woman conceives. As a mother she is another person than the woman without child. She carries the fruit of the night nine months long in her body. Something grows. Something grows into her life that never again departs from it. She is a mother. She is and remains a mother even though her child dies, though all her children die. For at one time she carried the child under her heart. And it does not go out of her heart ever again. Not even when it is dead. All this the man does not know; he knows nothing.
>
> *Birth,* David Meltzer

During pregnancy in particular, her body image, confidence in her sexual attractiveness and her sense of identity as a woman-person in the outer world are the focus of many conflicts throughout the nine months.

In the last three months, there are the joyful, practical tasks of preparation for the birth itself and the baby's arrival: attending childbirth classes, perhaps moving to larger quarters, lining a bassinet, painting a room. Underlying the outward-directed tasks is the necessary accompanying emotional preparation that goes on at the same time in unconscious forms—in dreams and fantasies working just below the daily level of consciousness. She has learned patience, an important quality for motherhood. The nine months of pregnancy have tested her. Often during those months nothing seems to be happening. She has been learning about nurturing and about caretaking as she carries her baby inside her.

As the actual birth approaches, emotions intensify. The pregnant couple is as close to the presence of life as to the possibility of death. In addition, the birth itself may have powerful sexual overtones reminiscent of the "letting go" and fear of death in orgasm. Women and men may find themselves suspended on an uncomfortable edge. Actor Donald Sutherland has vivid memories of the birth of his two children, at which he assisted:

> They were the best two days of my life. It is a very sexual thing to be right there when your child is being born. You just want to make love. It's as simple as that. But I don't plan on having any more children. In a strange way, seeing the two kids born was like psychologically participating in my own death...and I don't want to feel that again. It was like a part of me was cut away to give birth to a new life.
>
> *San Francisco Chronicle*
> September 30, 1979

We are unused to perceiving or talking about the sexuality of birth. As a holdover from Victorian attitudes, it has been a taboo subject. Only recently have women begun to share openly their feelings of pleasure and sexual arousal during birth and nursing. Acknowledging these natural feelings can increase the mutual pleasure and well-being of mother and child. Mr. Sutherland's description of his reaction to the births of his children is a fascinating illustration of the complex emotions birth can evoke in fathers, too—a sense of mortality, coupled with heightened sexuality. Indeed, the parents who are bringing life into the world may themselves feel an intensified sense of *being alive*.

During the pregnant year, as a man becomes a father, he may feel:

- Things will never be the same again.

- She'll love the baby more than me. I'll be jealous.

- She won't desire me again.

- I won't be a good father.

- Nothing I do satisfies her. It's never enough.

- I'm not sure I even want a kid.

- We made a baby!

- Her full breasts and her round belly turn me on.

- I can't understand the feelings she describes.

- I'll never be as important to the baby as she is.

- I envy her ability to create a person in her body.

- At least I make the money decisions around here.

- I love her sexual energy.

- I feel trapped.

- I feel left out, rejected. Who am I anyway? I need to feel attractive and special to someone.

- I can't wait to show off my kid.

- I'm afraid she won't be able to stand the pain. What if she screams for drugs?

- I won't be able to make enough money for all of us.

- I'm afraid she'll die.

- I don't want to end up as a diaper changer. It's demeaning.

- Now there will never be enough time for me.

- This is more important than anything else I've ever done.

- This baby will make such a difference in my life and relationship.

Until recently, most books on the pregnant years mentioned the father as the donor of the sperm on page one and promptly dismissed him. Some anthropologists say fatherhood is a social construct. Parenthood is now viewed as a social partnership. In a family where both partners work and each contributes to the family livelihood, a more realistic allocation of household responsibilities also needs to be shared. And even though it is still a bumpy partnership, it is progressing into a new kind of relating and sharing of social responsibility. The situation is changing, fortunately for everyone's benefit. Fathers are becoming more involved in the emotional preparation for parenthood as well. Although they have recently been encouraged to participate actively at the time of labor and delivery, little attention has been focused on their emotional needs during the year preceding the baby's birth. Many new books written by fathers are helping to adjust this imbalance. If we can tap the psychological resources of the father, says California psychiatrist Dr. Arthur Colman, he can be a deep well of support. However, in order to do that we must understand and meet his needs. In the last decades, researchers have been studying attitudes of expectant fathers and mapping the psychological stages that men pass through during the pregnant year.

Dr. James Herzog, a psychiatrist at the Harvard Medical School Children's Hospital and Judge Baker Children's Center in Brookline, Massachusetts, shows us that patterns of psychological experience in expectant fathers are as mappable as those of expectant mothers. These stages are not keyed to predictable physiological changes in men's bodies, but they are present and observable. We simply have never taken formal notice of these changes. Despite the fact that all men may not exhibit them to the same degree, "certain themes, feelings and concerns" repeat themselves across the pregnant months and are related to those of their partners. All men, however, are not in touch with their feelings to the same degree. Fathers in Herzog's study who were most aware of their own feelings about the pregnancy were those who were most attuned or sympathetic to their partners' intense feelings. The deeper the intimacy and commitment between partners, the easier it was for a man to fully participate in the changes that pregnancy brings. In couples where intimacy and commitment were weaker, concerns and fantasies about fathering become blurred or nonexistent. Furthermore, the origins of a father-to-be's nurturing behavior appear to go back to a man's own childhood and the nurturing he received.

The most empathetic fathers in Herzog's study spoke of the difference between simply having sex and "making a baby." When the conception was confirmed, these men were delighted: "Making the kid was a high," "We felt an inner glow," "I've got the cock that made her pregnant . . . my seed is sown." One man felt it gave him a reason for being. All were pleased with their potency and excited by the idea of creating a new life. The couples whose relationships were not as close, in contrast, did not plan the conception together, and in fact, some of these women chose not to share the news of their pregnant state for a while.

"Pregnancy is hard for men," says Jack Heinowitz in *Pregnant Fathers*. The father's life is transforming in subtle ways also. In Western societies, boys are not encouraged to express their deep feelings. "Keep your chin up," "Don't cry," "Be a man," "Be rational," we say. We teach them by words and example to deny and even to disparage their feelings. It is of more value to be strong, invulnerable, competitive. Parents, teachers, peers collude in maintaining this double standard for boys and girls. It is no wonder that fathers and sons are less apt to share in the intimate way that mothers and daughters do, even mothers and sons.

It's more culturally acceptable and easier for fathers to share their feelings with their daughters than their sons. It's an obvious outcome of the way we raise our sons.

Nor do we prepare boys to become family members and fathers. Girls, however, are expected and encouraged to play house, love their babydolls, help with their siblings, babysit with neighbors' children, cook, do laundry.

This double standard is a strand of the subliminal denial and belittlement of family values that women feel so acutely in the society and accounts for some of the stress felt between the sexes. Loss of communication, lack of shared values, insufficient emphasis on emotional and practical skills in family life can be attributed to the way we are raising our children in this society. A divorce rate in the 90's that is close to fifty percent may be the direct consequence of this value crisis in our society.

Societal attitudes impress us with the primary role of the mother. A mother's role is biological, her knowledge of motherhood and nurturing inborn. So goes the conventional wisdom. It's so easy, therefore, for an expectant father to feel his role is secondary. Lack of confidence, awkwardness, and confusion about his own role is an obvious consequence. His own father may have been absent as he was growing up, so it is by example and through cultural mythology that he may move aside during pregnancy, birth and the early infancy of his child.

Fathers resent being left out. Most want to be involved, but our societal attitudes and training don't prepare them for this important period in their lives. Many men have little experience with expressing the elusive feelings that this period of volatility arouses. Some men make the transition easily, but most feel awkward, detached, less communicative. And yet, the support a father-to-be can provide in confronting feelings of ambivalence—his own and his partner's—about the pregnancy is profoundly important to the well-being of the family.

Toward the end of the first trimester, the fathers who were most involved reported that their fantasies during lovemaking changed; that they experienced a shift in their inner life. Indeed, reports Herzog, it was through their sexual activity that they got in touch with their conflicts and feelings about caretaking and moved to a deeper understanding of their masculinity.

In Herzog's study, the sex lives of many men improved after their partners conceived. They not only wanted to be more loving toward their partners but they were able to ask them for love more easily, although some women don't feel too interested in the first trimester. For some, odd fantasies emerged during lovemaking. For example, there was a feeling of "refertilizing the pregnancy." Not only were they giving to the mother but to the baby as well. Some imagined they were "the breast" or "huge bottles of milk." One remarked, "They need more and I have it to give." For some fathers, it was a pleasure to have these new feelings; others felt irritation and concern about their capacity to meet the increased sexual demands. Or they themselves felt less desire because of their partner's body changes, or felt they were intruding into an already occupied body. One father in my group spoke of the sexual rejection he felt in the first few months and how he wanted to give his partner the same treatment when she got turned on again in the second trimester. When he spoke to other fathers, he realized he should not have taken it so personally.

Some men may feel responsible for making their partner pregnant and therefore are the cause of her discomfort. They may be very solicitous in the early pregnancy and ignore their own feelings of displacement as a result.

Some of the fathers were preoccupied with getting nurtured through sexual activity and often felt deprived, especially as their partner's interest declined in the later months. Just as pregnant women need more love and affection, so the men also may need extra evidence that they are still loved and desired. This is an important issue to be dealt with.

Expectant fathers also go through a spectrum of sexual fantasies and feelings of their own during this period. Watching his partner's body change and grow, month by month, provides dramatic proof to the expectant father that an irreversible transformation is taking place. A women's visible fertility may create many conflicting reactions in her partner: jealousy over her natural lifegiving productivity, fear of the Madonna she has become (and guilt at desiring a virginal Madonna figure), concern about entering her "already-occupied" body. Depending on his own background and self-esteem, this may temporarily wreak sexual havoc with his potency and his feelings of adequacy. Whether he turns to another woman for reassurance and sex or only thinks about doing so, his neediness may make him feel both guilty and resentful at the same time. This creates distance and tension just when a couple needs to be most supportive of each other. On the positive side, a man may also be drawn into a nurturing role and become a thoughtful caretaker of his partner and of the developing baby. This, too, however, may have its complications, for his new gentler caretaking impulses may frighten him, since his experience as a male in this culture has probably not encouraged development of this aspect of himself.

In mid-pregnancy, a man who is empathetic with his partner's experience may be far more conscious of his own emotions. Manifestations of *couvade* symptoms were shown by virtually everyone in Herzog's study. The *couvade* is such a fascinating phenomenon that it is worth examining in some detail. It is a psychosomatic expression of a psychological need that has only recently been rediscovered.

Couvade, derived from the old French word *couver* meaning to brood or to hatch, is a folk tradition that has been practiced with many variations in many parts of the world, and is of two types: 1) the father's imitation of the mother's role during and after childbirth, and 2) the subjection of the father to various dietary restrictions and to other privations and duties, often unpleasant, in order to protect the mother and baby from evil. Reports of the *couvade* date back to Herodotus, who discovered it in Africa, and to Marco Polo, who encountered it in ancient China.

The custom of couvade shows up in many societies today. No one seems to know its origin or to understand its meaning fully. One mythical version of the origin of the couvade, according to feminist author Helen Diner, is an Irish legend that tells of the pregnant wife of Crunniuc, who was forced to run a race against horses. Immediately after winning, she gave birth to twins. In the agonies of her birth pangs, she condemned all men who heard her cries to suffer the pains of childbirth for four days and five nights. The curse carried through nine generations.

Many other theories exist about the origin of couvade. Some think the custom arose to help the father identify with the new child and to accept responsibility for it. Since it is practiced almost exclusively in matriarchal societies, it may have been created to indicate that the act of birth is far more important than the act of insemination, and that it is only through the ritualized enactment of "giving birth" that the male becomes a father. Still other theories suggest the couvade may be an attempt to allow the father a more significant role through the psychodramatic technique of role reversal, or that it is an attempt to share the pain of childbirth through sympathetic magic.

Before, during, or after confinement, the father acts out the birth by lying in his bed, like his laboring wife. He moans, writhes, sobs and is nursed attentively. He accepts food restrictions for days or weeks before and after the birth occurs and is subject to the same customs as is the mother. For example, he is considered unclean after the birth until he has taken his first bath.

The practice has been observed recently by anthropologists in places as widespread as Siberia, the Malay Archipelago, in various countries in Africa and in Brazil and India. Somatic symptoms of couvade are reported in studies today in the United States. Often men express hidden feelings and will react physically to their partner's pregnancy. Some men notice their breasts swelling or experience a feeling of fullness. Sometimes, when a woman feels her partner is negative about the pregnancy, her attacks of nausea and fatigue may increase. On the other hand, if her partner is more strongly motivated towards parenthood and she is the more conflicted one, he may have the "morning sickness" and exhibit vicarious involvement through symptoms of pregnancy such as fatigue, dizziness, nausea, a swelling belly or breasts, food cravings, and even weight gain. These "couvade" responses are not at all uncommon.

In each society, the father's role is handled differently. In egalitarian societies, he is a valued and supportive participant, as in Polynesia, where attitudes and practices appear unburdened by complex ritual and sex roles are more equal. In such societies, there is no couvade. On the other hand, in male-dominated societies, where pregnancy is considered a dangerous time for the community at large and the pregnant woman is viewed as dirty and polluting, she is segregated and the father is restrained from the role of an involved supporter. Even in female-dominated societies, a pregnant woman will be supported by other women and fathers will be excluded. In these societies, the father will engage in couvade practices or participate vicariously.

In Java, it is believed that the husband's presence hastens delivery, since the child longs for its father, and therefore it is important that he attend the birth. Immediately after the birth, the mother and newborn baby bathe in the river, and thereafter the mother resumes her normal activities. The father, however, goes to bed, pretends to be sick and takes over the postpartum confinement while his wife prepares special food for him. (Couvade can have disadvantages for women!) It can become part of the negative attitude women inherit.

Anthropologist Margaret Mead's analysis of couvade practice links it to "birth envy" in males. The work of Melanie Klein, a psychoanalyst, speaks of male envy in relation to the creativity of women in childbirth. In fact, some psychologists say that a pregnant woman expects that envy and a dread of it creates anxiety in her. Bruno Bettleheim claims that a man who envies his partner's childbearing ability is not able to show sympathy for her. He expects, if not compels, her to resume her work immediately after childbirth although she may be exhausted and need to recuperate. The man, says Bettleheim, as husband and father, is permitted to rest. Instead of sympathy, emphasizes Bettleheim, the father insists on the special care for himself that would be appreciated by her but that he denies her. Bettleheim concludes that the expression of birth envy is less likely in a male-dominated society. He suggests that both male initiation rites and couvade rituals are parallel to a woman's childbirth rituals.

There are many other psychological phenomena experienced by men during the second trimester. During the middle period of the pregnancy, men often relive a childhood stage involving the hermaphroditic fantasy in which a boy believes he can both fertilize and bear a child. Colman reports that expectant fathers' dreams are filled with images of bearing and delivering babies. The appearances of these images in dreams, rather than being embarrassing, is a healthy sign that men are acknowledging their envy of a woman's capacity to conceive and nurture a new being within her body. In mythology, Zeus, in his envy of Athena's ability to procreate, consumes her, hoping to incorporate this creative capacity. Just as for women, if these often unconscious feelings are not dealt with by expectant fathers during pregnancy, they can reemerge at a later time in negative ways.

During the second trimester, men begin to perceive themselves as playing dual sexual roles. In Herzog's studies, fathers who were most intimate with their partners wanted to play at being both male and female. Many empathetic fathers, in fact, introduced variations in their lovemaking that allowed them to "feel penetrated at the same time that they were penetrating." These men felt that sexual activity made the baby happy and healthy. Others were either concerned that they might hurt the baby during sex, or that "the baby might bite." When a couple's personal relationship was warm and open, most men felt that the sexual relationship reflected this and was equally good. Toward the end of the pregnancy, reactions might be similar to that of one man who felt the mother's body was a "house" for the baby, which he could not enter.

Some men find the swelling belly to be sensual, a turn-on; others feel embarrassed and put off by the physical changes in their partner's body and will avert their eyes. This awkwardness stemming from their own backgrounds, can create personal distance. However, expectant mothers who feel unattractive and become jealous during pregnancy may find it reassuring to know that men, by and large, are more pleased by their partner's pregnant body than the women themselves are.

Some men unconsciously identify with the baby and the time they themselves were growing inside their mother's body, and may feel threatened. Others have been conditioned to consider the pregnant body unerotic. Women themselves may transmit this message because of the negative image they've encountered in the media.

This whole complex of psychosexual feelings is the harbinger of important change. What follows in mid-pregnancy, for men as well as for women, is an increased pressure to resolve one's relationship to one's own parents. This urge arises even if not recognized or acted on.

Interestingly, Herzog found that just as expectant mothers need to rework previous conflicts and unresolved feelings with the parent of the same sex, so too expectant fathers need to work out aspects of their own father-son relationship. Previous conflicts and tension come into play, particularly in relation to a man's own father.

The prospect of parenthood brings mother- and father-to-be into intimate contact with the life cycle. A need to reconnect with one's own father is one of the patterns of this time. Fathers-to-be need a father to lean on, and to learn from. They recall their father's behavior in their own childhood and want to adjust their own in relation to it:

> "My father walked away when emotions got hot in our family with us kids or with my mom. I want to be there and be a presence."

They want advice, modeling; they want to know what it means to be a man, a father/person in the continuum of their own family. It appears to be one of the necessary psychological steps toward achieving maturity and understanding the commitment and permanence inherent in the situation.

The Harvard study showed that a father involved in the pregnancy attempted to resolve issues with his father, often with his wife's help. Although these attempts were not always completely successful, relations improved as a result of the effort. Men who were least successful in breaking through these old barriers had the most difficult time during the second half of the pregnancy. Most knew that the process was important in some way. "How I hook up with my old man determines how the kid will hook up with me." It is as if men, like women, are symbolically and specifically trying to make a developmental leap from being the child of their fathers to becoming fathers to their child.

Other researchers stress a different aspect of a father's desire to fully participate—for there is nothing comparable they can do. It *is* an opportunity, however, for men to get in touch with their feminine nature, that is, with the receptive side of their nature, and to experience it and be able to express their feelings. The pregnant year for a prospective father too can be viewed as a demonstration of the interaction of opposites in the universe—a time to understand one's own androgynous nature.

Our culture stresses independence and performance for boys at an early age. They are told not to cry, not to show weakness, not to be vulnerable. It's not OK to express feelings. Being needy is not masculine. Sensitivity is mocked—even punishable, sometimes violently. Boys grow up in a rough and tumble, competitive world. These boys grow into men who feel they must solve their own emotional problems or be considered unmanly. Their sisters, on the other hand, are encouraged to cuddle, hug, play house, make close and intimate connections with family and friends.

It's clearly a double standard. And as adolescents and adults, we all suffer from this social template. Therefore, it is understandable that when an adult man moves into close and intimate connection with a woman, it is threatening to have a baby intrude into the safe, close relationship they have created.

There are many psychological strands. Some expectant fathers become competitive with their partners, provoked by unresolved feelings of sibling rivalry with the unborn baby, first initiated at the birth of their own brothers or sisters. This may also happen when men become partners with women in any situation, such as a business partnership. There may also be residual memories of their own sojourn in the womb and the separation at birth from their own mothers. Just as pregnant women relive feelings from their own birth and their childhood, so may fathers-to-be. The emotional swings and intensity of the pregnant months may also release in them unresolved issues from their childhood—feelings of abandonment or rejection, grief for a lost parent, feelings of dependency, or loss of self-esteem. The concerns are often subliminal. Dr. T. Berry Brazelton observes that a father-to-be's protective feelings about his partner may mask his own doubts and confusion. He may ask himself, says Brazelton, "Do I really want her to have my baby? Will she be a good enough mother? Unreasonably, he too, is looking for perfection. Because of the importance of the baby to him, he begins to wish for his own mother to be nurturing that child. The question about her competence really covers up questions about himself."

For the independent self-sufficient man, there may be a feeling of being swamped by the emotional intensity of a suddenly needy mother-to-be. He may feel trapped and withdraw, unable to be present for her. He may feel he has to handle his feelings and fears without her help. What to do? What gives her emotional relief may make him quite uncomfortable. Does he keep a stiff upper lip and bury his feelings? He may feel his partner's vulnerability and not want to turn to her for support. For some men who are used to being center stage, it is unfamiliar to take second place. They have been dethroned. They may feel quite isolated. A man may find that these and other primitive fears are hard to assimilate into the rational context in which he has functioned during his life up to this time.

Many men move on to the third trimester of the pregnancy with concerns and feelings that are similar to their partner's. They too experience the mystery and wonderment surrounding the awesome event—a process that is larger than themselves or any one person—and know that it is beyond their ability to control. They too become more concerned with practical matters, realizing that it is a time to get one's house in order, both literally and figuratively. Men become interested in how others cope; how others raise their children. They may observe and evaluate other men's performance as fathers-to-be and as fathers. A caretaking sensibility emerges for these men.

They begin to think about the birth itself and want to participate fully, as did the fathers in my group:

"I'm going to be there at the birth and for the first weeks after even if my boss doesn't like it. I'm not going to get cheated out of getting to know my baby from the start."

It is important for men to bond with their babies—for the baby and each member of the family.

Intrusive fantasies lessen with the decline of sexual activity. Some couples are sexually active until the birth. Physicians recommend various times for ceasing intercourse—anywhere from two to eight weeks or until the membranes rupture. There seems no clear cut wisdom. Orgasm in a pregnant woman does not initiate labor normally before term. When the baby is due it might. And there is no greater likelihood that a healthy couple will develop an infection during pregnancy than any other period. Doctors do restrict intercourse when there is bleeding, when the amniotic sac ruptures or when there is fear of the baby being born prematurely. Lovemaking and the intimacy it produces is a positive element during this changing time. Each couple finds its own way.

As the end of the pregnancy draws near, an outer-directed view replaces the absorption with the inner exploration of previous months. "It's out of my hands. I've done what I could. Now nature has to take its course."

It seemed to me that the mythic themes of mystery and wonderment that appear in every culture were reiterated over and over in Herzog's study and in my workshops. The spectrum varied from an emphasis on the sublime (meaning inspiring awe), or below the threshold of conscious perception to fear of death. Men began to sense the transpersonal dimensions of the experience of creation. Opening up to deeper feelings, many men considered their own mortality and the fragility of life. There were dreams of death—his own, his partner's, his child's. As he grappled with a more profound sense of responsibility for the creation of life and its nurture, he too became conscious of the cycle of life and death, just as Campbell reports.

There also emerges in fathers a more defined sense of the differences between male and female roles. And with it comes a new and deeper appreciation of their value as a person who goes out into the world, and conversely a new respect for the natural bond between mother and child. There emerges a clearer view of his role as the male person in the family.

Campbell speaks of the mythical father archetype's concern with the social order and social character of the child. A father realizes that he may be the most important provider, if not the sole one, for a period of time. He may become increasingly interested in community and world politics, environmental issues and education as he thinks about the future of his child. There may be more involvement in the outcome of these issues. Just as for women, these changes present an opportunity for growth. Implicit in the changes is an opportunity to see life through a wider lens, one that encompasses more of life.

Not surprisingly, taking into consideration cultural conditioning, the psychological and social dynamics of pregnancy appear to be different for men and women. Reactions will vary, of course, reflecting upbringing, adult personality and individual circumstances. For a man in particular, since his psychological state during this period is not linked to metabolic changes, his experience and involvement will be more directly related to his personal history, his past difficulties, the way he has previously resolved conflicts, and his psychological openness.

Anxiety seems to be a distinct part of pregnancy. There are so many issues: from the deepest metaphysical ones about the joy of creating new life to the fear of the psychological and social changes taking place, to the practical biological and financial concerns.

Pregnancy, especially the first time, is a profound and often overwhelming experience for most women and men. All that a woman knows and trusts about herself and her life is called into question daily, in fact, many times each day for nine months! In turn, her partner is sharing her concerns, as well as having to cope with his own changes. Unskilled at expressing feelings, he may be overwhelmed by the flood of emotions—his own and his partner's. They are asked to be especially understanding, empathetic and nurturing to each other. Being a nurturer is not a role men are raised to fill. For some, it's a big leap all at once. A man feels that he too, is in need of empathy and understanding for the important shifts that he is experiencing. And what he is experiencing is very different from what his partner is experiencing, since he is not pregnant and will not give birth. It's equally important for him to move through this rite of passage with a new sense of himself as it is for a woman—confronting his fears, his vulnerability and the changes that are so integral a part of the process.

A father-to-be may feel he will be evaluated on everything he does, as if he is being tested. An uncomfortable feeling. There are no rules to follow—just good clear thinking, intuition and sensitivity. Listening and just being there helps too, as does good open communication with one's partner and other men. And, of course, giving and receiving quantities of love and affection does a world of good.

Rather than going it alone in confusion, family and group support enable a prospective father to share his concerns with others going through the same process. Support is especially needed to work out inner and partner-related conflicts.

The third trimester is a time of profound change for everyone. If there are issues to be worked on, now is the time to confront them. A counselor can be found to help if needed. It has been demonstrated that problems can be dealt with more effectively during this period. Mutual support is necessary. In a group, one can share emotions, express positive feelings about oneself and this passage, and also work through feelings of fear, frustration, anger, or helplessness. It *is* a time of opportunity, for new learning and growth. Groups can be a rich source of support in loosening psychological knots.

The Seed

Lie on the floor; find a comfortable position; uncross your arms and legs so your energy can flow through your body.... Gently close your eyes and imagine a fluffy white cloud. Relax into your cloud,... sink deeper and deeper and even deeper into its softness.... Take a deep breath and let it go. As thoughts of your busy day intrude, allow them to drift away with an exhaled breath and bring your attention back to your breathing. Breathe gently, inhale and exhale, allowing your breath to take your tension away.... Relax, becoming lighter and lighter until you feel you are floating weightlessly, just like your baby.

Imagine a seed, a tiny seed resting in the palm of your hand. It is whole, pregnant with potential. It will become what it is meant to be—a flaming poppy, a velvet rose, a plump pear. Within this fertilized seed is knowledge of all that has gone before and a blueprint of what it will become. It knows just how to grow.... It will unfold, sprout, flower and fruit.

Within the womb is your seed unfolding, growing; within your seed is the knowledge of all that has gone before and a blueprint of what it will become. First this baby was a thought, then an expression of your love, and now it is an extension of your life. Be the sun and the moon to your baby and nurture it with your love. Trust what is happening. Be in tune with nature's process: all is going according to plan, the natural plan of life. Just as the sun warms the earth and energy to grow, so does your love give your baby energy to grow. Consider now, as the music carries you along, the ways in which you can create the most welcoming environment for your baby in your daily life....

Come back to this room now: feel the floor beneath you, massage your back against it, listen to the sounds in the room, take a deep breath and stretch. When you are ready, open your eyes and take in the entire room. Remember your experience and share it with your partner.

4

LOOSENING THE KNOTS: THE GROUP EXPERIENCE

Many people in different parts of the world entertain a strong objection to having any knot about their person at certain critical seasons, particularly childbirth, marriage and death. The Lapps think that a lying-in woman should have no knots on her garments, because a knot would have the effect of making the delivery difficult and painful. In the East Indies, this superstition is extended to the whole time of pregnancy; the people believe that if a pregnant woman were to tie knots, or braids, or make anything fast, the child would thereby be constricted or the woman herself be "tied up" when her time came. Nay, some of them enforce the observance of the rule on the father as well as the mother of the unborn child.

In all these cases the idea seems to be that the tying of a knot, would, as they say in the East Indies, "tie up" the woman, in other words, impede and perhaps prevent her delivery, or delay her convalescence after the birth.

In the island of Saghalien, when a woman is in labor, her husband undoes everything that can be undone. He loosens the plaits of his hair and the laces of his shoes. Then he unties whatever is tied in the house or its vicinity. In the courtyard, he takes the axe out of the log in which it is stuck; he unfastens the boat, if it is moored to a tree; he withdraws the cartridges from his gun, and the arrows from his crossbow.

The same train of thought underlies a practice observed by some people of opening all locks, doors and so on, while a birth is taking place in the house. Among the Mandelings of Sumatra, the lids of all chests, boxes, pans and so forth are opened; and if this does not produce the desired effects, the anxious husband has to strike the projecting ends of some of the housebeams in order to loosen them; for they think that "everything must be loose and open to facilitate the delivery."

The Golden Bough, 1929, Sir James Frazer

In the birth workshops, I hoped to create a concerned and supportive extended family and an emotionally safe environment. Conscious of the baby who is at the center of this change of state, I felt we might share together the profound changes that were taking place in each couple's sense of themselves, and feelings about each other and the ways their behavior might affect their unborn child.

By availing ourselves of the extraordinary sensitivity caused by the hormonal changes of pregnancy, I hoped we might loosen the psychological knots and provide the support that is needed from the very beginning.

How was I to begin? I contacted couples through doctors, midwives, childbirth educators, friends, ads in *New York* Magazine and in the *Village Voice,* letting people know that I was conducting four-month-long workshops at no fee as part of my doctoral research on the psychological and social aspects of "the pregnant year."

Based on my growing understanding of the developmental implications of the pregnant year, I designed pregnancy support groups for men and women who wanted to explore their feelings during the childbearing year, and to make an emotional connection to their not-yet-born children. In a sense, we were engaging in a "prenatal bonding" ritual; although we could not hold and touch the babies, we could speak to them, fantasize about them, visualize their environment in the womb and ima ine how our lives were affecting their development. Couples could prepare for the next stage by making the transition to familyhood on a gradual basis rather than in one sudden plunge after labor and delivery.

As this book documents, these groups had enormous value for those who participated. Step by step, I describe our early attempts to develop these workshops, and I suggest specific ways in which others might make these groups a reality in their own community. Finally, I offer my vision of a birth center that would provide an environment in which babies could be born, and families could evolve in harmony with the parents' emotional needs and with the highest regard for the health and well-being of their baby.

At first, it was difficult to find people who were willing to spend the weekly time and make the required commitment over time. I wanted couples who would come once a week for four months or more; it was not to be a "drop-in" group. Finally, most group members were referred to me by friends or were people I encountered personally.

At times I despaired that the first group would never come together. Pregnant women I met were intrigued, but many said, "*I'd* love to, but *he'd* never do it," or "I don't have the time." I was determined to have fathers as well as mothers. At dinner parties I got to be a bore, always inquiring about pregnant friends. Ultimately, my tenacity paid off. Seven couples signed up for the first group. One came through a woman I met at a party. Not pregnant herself but fascinated, she sent her brother and his pregnant wife. One couple came through *Ms.* Magazine friends, another through a male friend who couldn't have been less interested in birth. Two were sent by sympathetic obstetricians. The final couple read the ad in the paper. Seven pregnant couples—people who never would have met each other if not drawn together by their common interest in exploring pregnancy and birth. I was delighted. Unfortunately, a week before the first session, two couples had to drop out.

Despite the tentative beginning, the workshops were launched. Five couples joined me for the first session of the four-month-long venture. Women and men who were moving through the complex changes of pregnancy and preparing themselves to become parents, gathered together once a week. Under my guidance, they searched for answers to questions that had never occurred to them before. Much later, when the members of the first group had given birth, other groups were organized, some meeting for many months, others for intensive weekends. The groups were usually small, numbering about ten men and women. This size allowed everyone to participate actively and yet was large enough to provide a variety of reactions and experience. In this chapter, I have combined the reactions of many groups who met each week for several months.

The couples who participated in these support groups were, in general, white, middle class, primarily professionals—artists, writers, lawyers, architects, nurses, teachers—people who were intrigued by, although not particularly conscious of, the feelings provoked by the pregnancy. What they had in common was an eagerness and a commitment to talking with others who were going through the same experience. There was a span of ages. Most of the couples were in their thirties, though a few were younger and some of the men were in their early forties. In the four-month-long support groups, all the couples were expecting their first child, but were at different stages of pregnancy. (One couple came even before they conceived, and one couple was having a second child.) In the groups that met only for one intense weekend, there was, generally, a mixture of first and second pregnancies. Most couples in all the groups chose "natural" or "prepared childbirth" as a method of delivery, committing themselves to participate jointly in prenatal training and all stages of labor and delivery. Some mothers were turned off by the idea of "natural childbirth." Instead, they were frankly eager to yield the responsibility of the delivery to their doctors, whom they had carefully chosen to make decisions for them. These women said they didn't care whether or not they were "knocked out" by drugs. Their attitude often changed, however, during the course of the workshop. In the last six weeks of their pregnancies, all of the couples were involved in other prenatal classes whose major focus was on preparation for labor and delivery *per se*.

I made it clear that my major interest and expertise were not in the obstetrical or medical aspects of birth, but rather in the psychological process taking place. I hoped the group experience would be a source of education, so that they could make informed choices about the kind of delivery they hoped to have—hospital or home, with or without anesthesia, etc. As the groups progressed, I would make clear my own preferences, and share my own experiences—details of my birth, and of the births of my three children. We all felt a strong sense of excitement as we embarked on the journey of exploring aspects of pregnancy that have been neglected or minimized in contemporary Western society. What began for me as an interest in defining what might be an optimum physical environment for giving birth developed into a conviction that the emotional and physical aspects of pregnancy and birth are inseparable.

At the beginning I conducted the groups alone; in the subsequent groups I worked with a male co-leader. One of the co-leaders was a physician, a father of four, whose practice of internal medicine was based on holistic principles. He had experience in mind-body therapies, such as bioenergetics, and in group techniques, and was especially interested in how family interactions affect psychological and physical health. Best of all, he was warm, loving and a sensitive listener. He was as enthusiastic as I, welcoming the opportunity to work with a normal, healthy life transition.

In the group setting, we hoped to create:

- a safe place to raise questions and explore feelings— including expectations and fears;

- an environment in which each person could feel loved, trusted and valued;

- a supportive nonclinical environment in which parents-to-be shared their concerns with others moving through the same experience;

- ways to facilitate verbal and nonverbal communication in the couple relationship;

- insight and confidence in making personal decisions;

- tools, skills, information with which to design the birth experience;

- an atmosphere of celebration and joy.

The sessions developed in both unstructured and structured ways. I used explorative and supportive techniques that might help to make pregnancy a time of personal growth for each parent—as individuals, as a couple and as a part of a three-some, the developing family unit. I also used awareness techniques that have been developed in the West over the past several decades, as well as ancient Eastern ones. Many I myself improvised as the group progressed. These exercises helped to bring to conscious awareness intense feelings and emotions, such as confusion, tenderness, ambivalence and dependency. When possible, I initiated the workshop with a two-day session held over a weekend, with couples returning home at night.

At the beginning of each session, I found it helpful to start with a warm-up exercise, which effectively served to evoke concerns that had accumulated during the day. They also helped to focus on difficulties arising out of the pregnancy. Sometimes exercises were chosen to elicit feelings related to a particular theme. As trust developed in the group, so did spontaneity and expansiveness, and we were able to work in unstructured ways as well, allowing concerns to emerge spontaneously. Often a dramatic problem that had developed for one or another of the couples during the course of the week was used to highlight the issue and thereby gain insight. For example, a man coming home from work would expect the cheerful attention he received before pregnancy; instead, he might find his partner moody, withdrawn, self-absorbed, or in need of emotional comforting. This discrepancy in their mutual needs could create feelings of rejection and explosive tension if what was happening wasn't understood in a larger context. By playing each other's roles and acting out a typical incident, each partner could gain insight into the other's point of view. Group members observed the couple's behavior and pointed out unconscious behavior patterns. Since the workshop dealt with the shared concerns of pregnancy, problems discussed by one couple usually had significance for others.

* * * *

On a warm autumn Saturday in September 1972, my first group met at my home at ten in the morning for the first day of a two-day session. We gathered in the sunny living room of my garden apartment in New York City's Greenwich Village. We introduced ourselves, and talked about our expectations—positive and negative—for the group. I spoke of the many things that I hoped we could explore together, that I hoped to learn along with them and that although I had a vague agenda, it was to be their group. I wanted them to feel empowered not infantalized. I hoped the group would be responsive to their needs and their wishes would prevail. We had a preliminary discussion about time, schedules and commitment—details that in themselves are part of the process. I had to struggle with my own hopes, fears and expectations, along with everyone else. The couples were:

- Elene, a social worker, three months pregnant
- Dick, an architect
- Rachel, a homemaker, not yet pregnant
- Alan, a resident in internal medicine
- Amy, a weaver, four months pregnant
- Don, an economist
- Ria, a nursing student, four months pregnant
- Eric, a teacher
- Anne, a management consultant, two months pregnant
  Sam, an airlines executive

Interestingly, as each couple briefly described themselves, no one mentioned their occupation. For the time being, at least, they were willing to simply identify with parenthood. Even

Rachel and Alan, who had not yet conceived, chose that category. Positive reinforcement from the start. Encouraged by me, this couple had joined the group hoping that pregnancy might be "catching." They had tried everything else: she had been tested, he had been tested; they'd been through it all. We speculated that by focusing on the psychological process, the long-hoped-for conception might occur. It did some months later.

As we continued that morning, I suggested that each person keep a journal in which feelings, dreams, or important events would be recorded. Since so many changes would take place it would be hard to recall them later if they were not written down.

I asked permission to videotape the sessions so that we would have a record for others. Several couples expressed concern that it would affect their ability to share intimately. Ria, for one, didn't want to be recorded for "posterity"; others weren't sure what they felt. The decision was postponed until the end of the evening. Later, they all agreed that it was fine, and we agreed to start taping the following week.

The first exercise I introduced was a trust-building exercise called a blind walk: Everyone closed his-her eyes and allowed him-herself to be guided wordlessly through the space, trusting their partners to take care of them. They could lead each other up or downstairs, sit their partners down, guide them through different sound, temperature, and touch experiences—outside and inside the house. Simple as it seems, it is a surprisingly powerful and meaningful experience for pregnant couples in this increasingly interdependent time in their relationship. Symbolically, it is especially meaningful for a pregnant woman, who is involved in an organic experience, to entrust her body to others to guide her through.

Each couple had a turn leading and being led by their spouse and then working with another partner. Afterward, we discussed the experience together, sharing what had been learned about levels of trust. Several members talked about how much more secure they had felt with their partner than with a stranger. Amy described the panic she felt as she was led around by a strange person; Don described the disorientation he felt when shifting light patterns penetrated his colored eyelids. Later that morning he realized how dependent he was on his partner in their life together, and how difficult it was for him to acknowledge it.

An exercise such as this one can provide unexpected insights into one's need for a secure, trusting relationship. Being able to depend on one's partner is an important foundation for being able to handle other relationships in pregnancy where trust is at stake: doctors, nurses, hospital personnel. The themes of trust and dependency recurred often during the four months we spent together. To all of us, it became apparent that during this vulnerable period each partner needs constant nurturing in order to expand and change. The relationship needs the same capacity to stretch as does the pregnant belly. Pregnant couples found that they had to be mother, father and family for each other. Often the demands made on each other were felt to be excessive. The group provided additional emotional support.

Understanding one's own sense of what a loving parent might be was useful. We worked through another exercise:

BECOMING A PARENT

Find a comfortable position...uncross your arms and legs...close your eyes and become still...if thoughts of your busy day intrude, let them drift away...focus your attention on your breathing...take a deep breath and let it go...with each breath tension drifts away...take another breath...imagine yourself as a vessel through which love flows...inhale...and exhale...feel yourself relaxing deeper and deeper until you are fully relaxed...now remember a person in your life who was a wonderful mother or father to you...remember the qualities in this person that makes them so special to you...now remember an occasion when you loved being mothered...loved being fathered...Let the music carry you back to one of those times and let yourself experience the feelings of that time and as you do, become aware of the qualities in yourself that will make you, too, a loving parent...

Begin to stir again...come back to the room gradually...even before you open your eyes remember what the room looked like...hear the sounds...sense the movement in the air...become aware of the floor beneath you...slowly open your eyes...and look around with a soft unfocused gaze...when you are ready, sit up and share your experience with your partner.

* * * *

After three hours of unfamiliar and stimulating interactions, everyone needed a break. We stopped to relax and share the potluck meal that everyone had brought. "Breaking bread" together seemed an appropriate ritual for the nurturing process of exploration that we were embarking on. It was also a chance to socialize on a more informal level.

Everyone gathered round the table in my country-style kitchen. The autumn sun filtered through the garden out back, creating golden stripes on polished floorboards. Graced with heavy rafters and a large fireplace, the kitchen had fed many families since it was built in 1835. Its warm environment enhanced our workshop. It was an atmosphere that could not have been achieved at a prenatal clinic. Although no one had specifically designated what should be brought to the pot luck, the bread, salads and casseroles all came together as a three-course meal. Have you ever noticed how often things work out when one doesn't try to maintain control? It was as if from the beginning of our first session the group became a functioning organism. It was a joy to see the pregnant women survey the food-laden table. The men also beamed in anticipation, but they weren't feasting for two. Being well fed and nurtured, however, increased everyone's feeling of well-being. Each couple brought food that was an expression of their life and attitudes: simple health food from one, complicated gourmet sauces from another. We were already learning about each other.

After lunch, we gathered again and I suggested another exercise.

MEDITATION ON BIRTH

In a room emptied of furniture, I asked everyone to lie down and form a mandala shaped like the spokes in a wheel, with heads touching in the middle of the circle, husbands and wives alternating as they lay on the floor. I began,

> Pay attention to your breathing. Simply allow its normal rhythm without controlling it. Relax more deeply with each breath—as it moves in and out, inhale and exhale—and with each breath let go of your thoughts, let them float by as you breathe out, let go of your persona, your profession, your attachments, just become aware of your breath connecting you to the universe.

After some minutes of stillness, I continued by guiding them back to the room and to their connection with each other. Each couple was asked to join hands and with their eyes still closed, to sense their partner's breathing rhythm and to breathe in unison with one another and with the baby in the womb.

> Get in touch with the rhythm you are now sharing, the rise and fall of joined breathing...and with the baby's rhythm...When you feel in synchrony with each other, begin to meditate on the word *Birth*. Allow your thoughts to arise and flow through your consciousness, let them come and go. Simply observe without trying to hold on to them, allow them to drift through...When you are ready, open your eyes.

* * * *

All of this took about twenty minutes. Quietly, still in meditative silence, we returned to the other room. Interestingly, some couples felt relaxed, chose new places to sit. However, they remained a pair sitting close together. Sometime later, when we discussed our seating patterns, couples became aware of how little time they had with each other during the week. They realized that it was not only for security in this unfamiliar situation that they chose to sit next to their partners, but in order to be able to be close and to touch.

> "We talked about what had happened that morning." Ria began: "I was aware of many new sensations in my body

> that I don't normally take time to sense...It has changed.
> Rather than feeling uncomfortable about that, as I normally
> do, I was really digging it...and then I began to picture the
> development of the baby. I was acutely aware that my baby
> isn't ready to be born yet. I can't explain how I know that, I
> just know it in a lot of ways. The baby and I seemed to
> understand about that."

As a result of our morning's work, Don was aware of how awed he was by pregnancy and birth:

> You know, no matter what we say about men and women
> and their individual part in producing a child, I am con-
> stantly awed by the wonder of it. Whatever you say about
> different societal attitudes towards birth over the centuries,
> giving birth is a power and a privilege. Something men are
> dwarfed by....I never consider that it's convenient for my
> wife to carry and bear our child, that it's wonderful and that
> I don't have that burden. I don't feel it's a burden at all. It's
> a mysterious process...maybe that's why I unconsciously
> step back from it because it's awesome and fearsome...pri-
> mordial. Maybe that's why I stare so much...as if you are
> the goddess, the Divine Mother...

His wife, Amy, found his reverent stares disconcerting; rather than feeling admired, she felt his gaze to be distancing and impersonal. "I feel too earthy and needy to be larger than life."

Other men also had a tendency to focus on the mythic aspects of motherhood:

> I thought about being born myself and about how we feel
> we all share that primal attachment to the mother. I felt
> identified with my baby and myself as baby and got to feel-
> ing quite sentimental about my own mother as goddess. Ye
> Gods, I've never thought of her in those terms before.

One man picked up on the contrast between men's and women's roles in childbearing:

Leni, I hear you suggesting that men envy women's ability to carry a child in their bodies. I don't feel that way at all. I feel I put the child there and I will have all the benefits of having a child without the burden of having to carry it around. So instead of feeling envy for her ability to make a child grow, I feel quite the opposite.

The group was momentarily silenced by the chauvinism of that remark.

The meditation was powerful for Rachel and Alan, who had not yet conceived. Full of anxiety and questions about pregnancy and birth and parenthood, they felt delighted to be part of the group in order to eliminate emotional barriers to a possible conception.

Rachel: Birth looms as such an overwhelming experience for me, I feel I might be swept away. The idea of the possible pain of labor and delivery terrifies me. I can't get past those spectres.

Before she met Alan, she'd had an abortion. Her guilt about that decision was still with her. During the morning exercise, her unresolved feelings about the abortion had been stirred up. Now, as she began to tell us the story, tears flooded down her face.

In talking about it with the group, Alan realized how much feeling he still had about it. Each of us was caught up in our own emotional response as we listened. Alan recalled the time when she had first told him about her abortion. It remained a highly charged issue between them, especially now during their unsuccessful attempts to conceive. The trust level in the group deepened as Rachel risked her vulnerable feelings so openly. Silence followed.

The group was getting used to each other. Amy talked about the abortion she'd had some years before. It had been very scary and badly handled by the clinic, so she had strong empathy for Rachel. She went on to say that the memory was pretty dim now.

I feel that's well behind me now. I was in touch with a sense of inadequacy when I was focusing on the exercise. I kept hearing myself say, "I'm still a kid, how can I be having a kid?" I hoped the baby wasn't listening.

Other reactions were voiced. Diverse feelings had been triggered by the exercise. Again and again in later sessions, I felt that the exercises were invaluable aids for bringing painful, repressed memories to the surface where they could be gently examined and correlated with present difficulties. Most often I didn't set a theme for any evening's discussion, and allowed instead the needs or mood of the group to determine what we dealt with. Exercises that I had designed to help couples work on different issues were modified to fit the moment. Often, highly volatile issues could best be dealt with by first participating in a group exercise in which no one was required to be analytical.

Feelings of anger, frustration, confusion—a whole spectrum of heightened sensitivities, awakened by the stress of the transitional period—arose and needed to be examined in a supportive environment.

Practical decision-making creates stress—questions of timing, readiness to begin a family, how many, how far apart. Can we afford it? What about our careers? Who gives up what and when?

Old childhood fantasies, anxieties and archetypal images that normally lay dormant in the subconscious rose to the surface of their everyday reality to trigger and unleash a whole Pandora's box of fears: fear of loss of control, of the unknown, dependency, rejection, incompetence—of death; death of one's self, of one's partner-provider, or the baby. It was clear that these themes did not arise only as discrete ideas, but were intertwined and interdependent themselves. Some themes were more resonant for one couple than another. For example, if, in one situation, a man did not give a woman enough appreciation for her developing pregnant body, she might tumble into despair. Another woman might not have any reaction. Financial considerations might plague one expectant father more than another or a sense of inadequacy frighten one woman while another felt confident. Old, lifelong patterns of acknowledgment—or lack of it—might be at the base of these responses.

One of the personal tasks assigned to group members was learning about their own biological births, about the circumstances and attitudes of their parents, siblings and relatives—whatever might throw light on conflicted and possibly even negative feelings about pregnancy and birth. The group, I felt, was a place in which experiences, possibly as traumatic as my own birth recollections, might be discussed in a supportive and explorative atmosphere.

As we met for three or four hours once a week over the months, couples relaxed, and, in most cases, began to develop a deeper level of intimacy with each other and with the group. As the session progressed during succeeding evenings, particular themes emerged in the group. Similar patterns were apparent in the groups that followed.

I usually started the evening with a meditation or relaxation exercise to allow everyone to come together and to let go of the day's activities. This might be followed by another exercise designed to catalyze feelings and help us to move to a deeper subjective level.

In the course of the workshops, we untangled many knotted strands of personal history which allowed a new self—a parent self—to evolve. Sometimes this happened through sudden "Ah, Ha!" insights, sometimes simply through the subtle realization that a certain stimulus no longer evoked a particular response. It seems to be true that one never quite knows how personal change will take place.

We moved along, swept forward by the forceful physiological changes the women were undergoing. While we were actually meeting, I didn't categorize or label our discussions, but in reviewing the sessions, it was clear that the classical themes of pregnancy arose again and again.

Ambivalence was a key issue early in everyone's pregnancy. Its intensity disappeared as the baby's actual presence became more apparent. And if not confronted in the early months, repressed ambivalence might be triggered by other issues.

Sometimes those ambivalent feelings reemerged in the eighth month as the baby's arrival became imminent.

At the beginning when the bulge was not yet apparent, pregnancy could either be kept a secret or announced with pride to all the world. Women dealt with it in quite different ways. Some preferred to become accustomed to the idea gradually, privately, slowly acknowledging the enormity of what was taking place deep within them. Often it was almost impossible to accept the reality of it all; as Elena put it:

> What surprised me was the intensity of the revulsion I occasionally felt when I considered the appearance of the fetus in books like Nilsson's *A Child Is Born*. I really didn't like the realization that *that* was inside me and moving about.

Even women who were motivated toward pregnancy entertained second thoughts. Often, though they had been eager to conceive, they still struggled against negative feelings during those first difficult weeks. And then, after an initial adjustment, pregnancy seemed quite natural and other matters quickly claimed their attention. After her initial reluctance, Elena began to respond to the life force within her. "It is like a tree that emerged from the ground and needed to be nourished."

Taking in and integrating the reality of the pregnancy may take longer for men since it is not happening to them physically.

> **Eric:** My thoughts and feelings are in an uproar. I know I'm supposed to feel excited but I don't. Maybe I'm just suppressing my fear. What if I hate being a father, tied down to the marriage and the kid—my freedom's gone.

Adjusting to the reality of the pregnancy and its future implications is a subtle and continuing task for both mother and father. Each has his or her own problems and joys with it.

> **Don:** Becoming pregnant was like growing up for real. I had to reaccess everything. My responsibilities, my values, my goals. Helping to create a new life really did it to me.

On one occasion, I asked the group whether this was a *planned* pregnancy and about their reaction when they learned the news; there was an embarrassed silence followed by nervous laughter.

Amy's reactions to her pregnancy were mixed. As a weaver, who had only recently quit her job to weave full-time, she was troubled by the ambivalence she felt and concerned that her unresolved emotions might harm the child.

> I was a little glad and a little sad. First of all I couldn't believe it. I was over thirty and had never conceived. All my friends had been having abortions for years. This is the first year of my life when I'm doing what I want to be doing and although Don is very sympathetic and I really want to have this baby, I'm resenting it, too.

It was a relief, she said, to admit it out loud.
One man admitted he hadn't been ready for fatherhood at all.

> I seriously considered an abortion for us, but now that I see my wife's belly, I realize it was outrageous.

And others said:

> **Elena:** Planned? It's hard to say...right now my fantasies are pretty scary sometimes. Whenever I'm feeling fearful or worried about what it's going to be like to be a mother or even whether I really want it, I start to feel guilty. That's when I imagine that the baby wants to get even with me...I feel it knows what I'm thinking.

> **Ed:** It was a toss-up for me. Was I glad? I like to be free-wheeling. Committing—marrying was a struggle, but now I find I'm enjoying the idea of having a family to come home to, a secure place with continuity. I'm really surprised.

> **Anne:** I can't believe it's really happening to me...that I'm pregnant, that we're going to have a child. Sam's delighted, I'm scared. It's a relief to know others have fears, too, that it happens with other people...that it's O.K. to have fears.

Maybe I can begin to share some of the warm pleasurable feelings, too.

Amy: So much is happening for me, it's hard to focus beyond it. I know I'm shutting Don out. It's hard to stay on top of it.

Ria and Eric's story leaked out gradually and was never fully revealed until after the baby was born, when Eric revealed to me that he'd been extremely ambivalent early in the pregnancy but afraid to reveal it.

I had trouble concentrating on work. I needed to spend more time by myself to process. I wasn't as excited as I was supposed to be. I was pretending I was.

Ria, on the other hand, dealt with issues more openly during the group:

Yesterday I went to visit a friend who has a six-year-old, a three-year-old and a four-month-old baby. It was great to hold the baby, I think that's why I headed for her house. I was also overwhelmed by the horrible sense of what it means to bring into one's house a little creature who can never again be left alone and is such an enormous and inescapable responsibility. I realized that I have chosen such a responsibility, and that I don't know what I have gotten myself and Eric into...I guess I feel a little more peaceful about all that but it isn't resolved yet.

Only much later, long after the births, when I asked people to reflect on their experiences in the group, did I discover the intensity of the feelings involved for Eric and Ria.

Often it was through journals kept during the workshops that people were able to express conflicts and emotional turmoil. Sometimes entries were read out loud. Usually, it was the women who wrote. Anne had started keeping a journal even before joining the group.

I feel trapped. Maybe an abortion. It's not happening to me. It's a movie and I'll play a part (simpering motherhood, cherubic smile) but I don't feel it. I'm numb. Next, I'm scared. What have we done? Dreams of death—my dear parents' death. One night, stark terror, nameless.

I haven't been able to completely shake the terror that I felt that night six-eight weeks ago, when I woke up in the middle of the night absolutely terrified in the depths of my being...pure terror, unlike anything I'd ever felt except maybe as a young child. Nothing Sam or anyone else could do could reach it. It reaches to the core of me.

Oh my God, there's nothing I can do, nothing you can do, nothing to be done. It's finally happening, it's happened. A baby! The dread—maybe it will happen—is replaced by certainty. Oh God, Oh Lord, there's nothing we can do, I can do.

Occasionally, I have little episodes of fear, rising from the solar plexus through chest to throat where I succeed in choking it off. Like when I heard Hal describing the research on care of infants just after birth. I don't want to hear about it. Or like when I am telling people I am pregnant. The same rising wave. Some of the fear escapes from my eyes.

And then after the first couple of sessions:

Sometimes I feel smug. I'll be sitting in a meeting at work and think, there's something very special happening and you all don't know what it's like.

Her later entries showed steady progress in accepting the pregnancy:

At Christmas, I pop out, begin to show. I start telling friends and office mates—a great relief not to have some secret, almost like a malignant disease! I relax more. I begin to let the positive feelings well up. Still some uncertainty but I'm getting grounded.

Lately, I've been asking myself why can't I take this motherhood thing in stride? Why does it seem so earth shattering? I'm going to be more mature, take it in stride.

Feeling anxious and expressing it can be overdone...I haven't expressed my competent side enough.

Sam is really delighted about the offspring (his drawing of skipping father with big heart which he drew in the group)...He doesn't show this very directly in the group; he stays at a philosophic conceptual level most of the time— but then seeing him in the group allows me to see that these joyful feelings are there for him, too. The nonverbal work helps our sharing. Sam's and mine.

We noticed symptoms of pregnancy such as nausea, swelling bellies and food cravings among some of the men in the group—classical couvade symptoms. One man had back pain for four months, beginning in the fifth month of his wife's pregnancy. He noted in his journal:

I thought I was going to be wheeled into the delivery room with Nancy. I joked about the serious pain in my back; it was so embarrassing. It seemed obvious it was connected to the baby. It struck me that it was like hiccoughing for two days straight before our wedding.

Another man told us that at his birth, his father developed shingles right afterwards. This meant that his mother and he had to remain in the hospital until a nurse could be found to take care of all of them at home. It meant a lot that his father shared his memories with him.

Many fathers in the group were awed by the developing pregnancy and felt distant from the experience. Some were able to acknowledge that they felt envious of their wives' biological role.

Dick: Sure, I'm jealous. Sure, I would like to carry a baby. It must be colossal of course, but there is the weight and the discomfort, and to feel this thing growing inside of me!

Alan: Men go around biologically unfulfilled in a way. Perhaps there is envy of the satisfaction that comes with completing certain biological life cycles. How many life cycles do men complete...just birth and death? Somehow ejaculation is not the same thing. I envy the stress a woman feels as she passes through the big event.

Eric: I was never consciously envious, though I have some friends who have gone through giving birth trips—pseudo-deliveries and pseudobirths...

I don't feel as if I had much responsibility in the creation of the baby. It's a little weird to me but then I say to myself ...who else is responsible?

Biological paternity was discussed very gingerly. It sounded so disloyal. But the subject did surface. The men discussed it abstractly. It was much easier than confronting their own doubts.

How could one know? Until the kid comes out and doesn't look like you. Nervous laughter followed by awkward silence.

In the midst of one such discussion, I suggested that it would be more effective if the men really tried to imagine what it would be like to be pregnant rather than talking about it so abstractly. We decided to perform the exercise called "Father's Fantasy of Being Pregnant." I asked them to stuff pillows under their shirts and sit in a circle in the middle of the room. The wives were delighted. After a moment or two of silence, I began to guide them into a fantasy of pregnancy. They sat with eyes closed, sensing their expanded shape, swollen with the life inside it.

Close your eyes. Breathe gently and naturally, allowing your breath to rise and fall without changing its rhythm. Feel your belly with your hands. Feel the roundness of it, the firmness of it, feel the pressure of the uterus against your chest and the bulge resting on your lap. Your belly has been growing gradually for the past months—you are seven months pregnant. You are feeling full and ripe. The baby is moving about inside you, kicking, turning, making its presence felt.

I asked them to speak when they felt the urge. It didn't take long for the words to come.

It's like having a nice companion with me, but I don't like having a big belly; it's getting in my way. It keeps me away from other people. I have a feeling of disfigurement. At first I just felt I had a pillow against my stomach and I felt silly, but then I thought what if I had to watch it grow slowly. I imagine I might feel some resentment about it. It's a tumor; I'm glad I can take the pillow out and put the whole thing away. I'm just as happy to let someone else carry it. How's yours?

* * * *

Dick: Great! We "women" are lucky. It allows us to keep in touch with the cosmos. I think my belly is a majestic thing, a fantastic thing. It is like a drum, this taut thing, full of life. I'm proud of this bulging belly, not at all disfigured. What's disfiguring? It's life!

After the exercise, Amy spoke:

I've always been glad to be on this side of it and felt sorry for men. I always wondered how they felt, so I'm relieved that they don't feel that they are missing a lot. Now I can be greedy about enjoying my pregnant state.

Leni: And might you want to go one step further and tell Don what you would like over and beyond being able to enjoy this state or what might help you get even more out of it?

Amy: I want you to appreciate me as a woman and really feel the life and the movement inside me all the time...It never seems to stop. I want you to feel the wonder of it the way I do and the beauty...and the beauty of my form, too. I want you to feel part of the whole thing. I want you to say to people..."Look, that's my wife carrying my kid."

Although most of the women loved their changing form, their productive interior, it brought with it continuing problems of self-image and feelings of intrusion. Early in the pregnancy, before the baby's movements were felt, Amy was sorting out the "I feel the bulge is me and yet not me" feelings. Later on, as Amy's form swelled, the pregnancy was undeniable, yet still hard to fully absorb on a deeper psychological level:

> Who am I in relation to this intruder who is taking over my body? It's a problem for me: I wake up in the night feeling outraged at this insistent being, this parasitic intruder inside my body.

Anne wrote in her journal during the first months:

> The knowing, from the first weeks, of the change of the activity and the presence, especially the presence. No longer a space but a form, an energy.
>
> Knowing, but at first not wanting to believe. And yet, hiding a Mona Lisa smile...
>
> I've touched the edge of time and space. I'm connected to it, the link is made.

> **Ria:** I caught a glimpse of myself in the mirror—the full-length mirror in the locker room at the pool at school—and I pulled my dress in to outline my belly. I still can't believe it's a baby, that I'm really pregnant as I've imagined being, as I've hoped I'd be, almost all my life.

> **Jean:** My father-in-law and I have bellies that meet, but he doesn't like me to point it out. The funniest thing about my changing shape is growing so big that I can't even see my feet when I look down. Since I know it's temporary, I play games about being a fat person and having a big belly.

Many were proud of their changing form and the new status it implied, and longed for everyone to notice.

> **Elene:** I feel I'm very beautiful to myself and Dick. I'm doting on that. I love my developing belly.

Some women worried about losing their appeal. An animated discussion developed around that issue one night. Feelings tumbled out.

> **Elena:** When a pregnant friend and I walk together on the street and catch a sight of our roly-poly reflections in the store windows, we go into gales of laughter like adolescents. But if our husbands laugh at our misshapen bodies, or our transient moods, it's another matter. We get quite depressed.

> **Amy:** I was thinking that you never see a pregnant pin-up. I've been looking at a lot of birth books—some of the pictures are so striking—the beauty and sensuality of the roundness. Sometimes when I shower, I just look at this big belly and love that it is there.

Elena persisted quietly:

> But sometimes I feel quite fat and ugly and I find myself watching other women's bodies. Do you have that problem? I find I go into a tailspin, afraid that Dick will stray away.
>
> This is the first time in my life that I've had some physical limitation and, of course, I realize it is indicative of the whole change of life-style.

Self-image, dependency, trust were all inextricably entangled in this transition from being a couple to becoming a family. These strands were woven back and forth through the workshop.

> **Amy:** What's so hard to face is my dependency as Don has withdrawn into himself; I realize painfully how much we do together normally and how much I count on that.

> **Beth:** After the struggle to be independent and autonomous, I was suddenly so vulnerable and dependent in every way. Fortunately, it never came out in resentment towards the baby. But it's causing a lot of tension between Nick and me.

In response to Beth's increasing and uncharacteristic neediness, Nick admitted he often found himself withholding the very
affection and nurturing that she needed to feel comforted or
turned-on sexually. When this happened, they would retire to
their corners in a tangle of confusion and misunderstanding.
Both would end up suffering.

There were repetitive themes underlying the conflicts that
arose between partners:

- Are you hearing me?

- Will you respond to me?

- Can I depend on you?

- Can I trust you?

For many men, it became difficult to handle the increased
demands and dependency, threatened as they were by their
own feelings of insecurity in anticipation of another person in
their lives. In the groups, they were encouraged to examine tensions as they arose, rather than withdrawing or keeping up a
good front.

> It's tough for me to feel rejected. I had a lot of that growing
> up. It's coming up again with Jane being so consumed by
> the baby. It's hard to admit but sometimes I find myself fan-
> tasizing a hot affair.

Some men take on more work, or hang out with their friends,
or even fantasize about having another sexual liaison in the face
of what feels like rejection. During pregnancy, they fear that the
closeness of the relationship will deteriorate.

One evening Elena and Dick arrived, furious at each other.
Most of the evening was devoted to clarifying what had happened to them since the last session of the group. It had started
over a simple thing. Elena had wanted Dick to go to a meeting
with her one night. He said no. She took it as a personal rejection. It became a matter of his attention to her.

> The following week Elena came back, looking radiant. It was so good to be able to work that problem out here. I think it was getting it out in a situation that was safe, with people who had similar concerns...that's been really helpful, because I felt good this week and I felt that Dick and I were good together this week. If we had a similar discussion at home it would have just...in fact, we have had similar discussions, and it didn't clarify anything. I don't think we always need people, but I think on that sticky issue we worked through, it was really helpful.

Making sure the men were included was an issue women didn't think about enough. The women needed ways to include their partners in the pregnancy. Cultural norms and their own awkwardness caused barriers. Since men don't have direct access to the child in the womb, they need a mate's generous help to begin early bonding with their child.

> Elena is very accepting of my involvement with the baby. I love stroking her belly and feeling a response from the baby. I have always played the flute so I picked that up again. It's a way I feel in touch. It makes us more of a family already.

Misunderstandings related to increased dependency were a major problem for most couples. Sometimes the conflict went like this:

> **Alan:** Reconnecting at the end of the day is a problem. When I come home, Rachel's been home all day; she wants to share her experience of the day—but even though I've come home, I'm still working—I want to complete some phone calls, make some notes...She wants to connect and I'm experiencing something else. I really feel pushed.

> **Rachel:** Sure you answer me, but I need something more from you—a reaction, for instance—I imagine something is going on in you, you're upset and not sharing it and I hesitate to say other things and it starts a whole spiral of angry behavior and missed signals.

Often, conflicts reflect patterns of unresolved behavior from childhood and the pregnant period becomes a time to confront it once again and work it through, often with more satisfying, conclusive results. I suggested that evening that Rachel and Alan try a Gestalt exercise called "I Resent." They were asked to sit opposite each other and trade resentments. Alan began.

> I resent it when you involve me the moment I walk in the door. I resent it when you want me to listen to the events of your day whether they were positive or a drag...

After a mechanical start, Alan warmed to the task; he poured out a long list of resentments, becoming more and more emotional as he progressed. Rachel was instructed to sit quietly and listen without responding. She then followed with her list of past and present grievances and resentments. Rachel expressed surprise at how familiar the resentments sounded, commenting, "I sound like my mother, for God's sake." It was a catharsis, to be sure, and also an opportunity to observe how one can project childhood resentments onto present circumstances.

> **Alan:** It's sure something to guard against in the future. I realize that if Rachel gives me space to unwind and get my head clear and then I still don't come around, or respond after a while, she sure has a valid complaint. Then I really have to acknowledge that negative behavior.

After they finished exchanging resentments, they spent time expressing the positive side of the same exercise called "I Appreciate," which works in a similar fashion. At the end of the exercise, they discussed how they might spend time together at the end of the work day, when each needed contact but might not be ready to talk. For instance, they considered as a homecoming ritual taking a bath together, massaging each other, or just lying quietly on the bed in each other's arms—gentle ways to be in touch, ways to sense rather than using words to explain their mood. They talked of including the unborn baby in their new homecoming ritual, and were pleased that the exercise had worked so well. For them, as for many of us, words tend to be such a habitual way of connecting that we forget the power of a tender exchange expressed through touch, and the importance of gentling one another.

After Rachel and Alan had resolved their differences, the group participated in "Hand Conversation," a nonverbal communication exercise. Partners stood opposite each other and grasped hands as if in meeting. They were limited to expressing themselves through their hands: feelings of pleasure, anger, impatience, or whatever was present. Afterward, we discussed the emotions the exercise evoked. Some people had been surprised by the way play had turned into aggression. Others found their connection very sensual.

The next week, Rachel reported that the "I Resent" exercise had really helped her to see Alan's point of view. Rachel said thoughtfully:

> If I tackle Alan at the door with either my enthusiasm or my neediness, I hear my inner voice saying "You've done it again!"

For most men, it was difficult to accompany their partners on the emotional roller coaster of pregnancy, since their hormones were not providing them with the same momentum.

> **Don:** It's not only that Amy's normal emotions are amplified, but I simply tune in to a different channel in life.
> Yes, I guess, I tune out because I feel so inadequate. I don't know how to even begin to be comforting, since I don't have any familiarity with such highs and lows.

But some expectant fathers were having an opposite experience:

> **John:** Recently, I felt as if I tapped a well spring inside me. I was always a stoic at movies, now I cry—can't believe it. It's as if the cork came out of my feelings.

Lovemaking, a form of intense, tender communication that might normally dissipate some of this distance, can itself become a source of misunderstanding and hurt feelings during pregnancy.

Some women in the groups became withdrawn, self-absorbed and turned-off sexually as the pregnancy advanced. Others felt passive and more dependent. They needed affection and cuddling more than sex. Jan, at eight months, said:

> I feel disinterested in sex but I'm worried about being indifferent and turned off. I'm afraid Peter will wander off and have an affair.

Elena had similar feelings:

> We need each other but in different ways. For instance, I want to be held and cuddled and Dick wants to have intercourse. It causes a lot of tension when we can't talk it through.

Ironically, whether women wanted less sex or more sex, they worried about their partners' responses to their new patterns. As one might expect, many women experienced a heightened interest during the early months, and often felt anxious about making too many demands on their husbands. Others felt confused by the simultaneous, competitive pull between the roles of wife, lover and mother. There was a continuing problem of learning to talk clearly about intensified needs and fears:

> **Don:** The first few months were awful for me. I wanted to be close. That meant sex. But Amy wanted none of it. It was tough!

> **Alan:** Underneath the disagreeableness we get into, is the question, "Why aren't you there for me?" followed by "Is this what's going to happen in the future?" It's the fear of that.

> **Rachel:** I'm thinking the same thing . . . "Am I going to be left with the kid all the time?"

> **Anne:** We still have problems asking for what we need but we're getting better. Practicing here in the group helps. I seem to be asking for more, at least that's what Sam says,

although I feel I'm still asking for the same old things—to be seen and heard. Maybe, the volume is just turned up now—Our professional lives have been quite separate. We have had different orbits for a long time, but now the pregnancy is bringing us more together, and I think the baby will do that even more.

Rachel: Why is a demand automatically a big awkward thing?

Alan: It is as if at times I am treated without personal respect, as though things were expected of me. I have to do it, it doesn't matter if I do it out of love or not, it just is expected.

In the groups, we found people had a safe place where they could risk being vulnerable in order to open up communication with their partners.

Beth: I've had a hard time this week and I realize I don't know how to ask Nick for help for my little-girl self. I don't know whether I'm asking for it for my wife-grown-up self or for my little-girl self. I want to say, "Please, Nick, protect me. I need you."

It's important that you let this little girl that's in me get protection because I never got it from my father... at least a sense of physical stroking and protection. My father never held me, he never stroked me, he never kissed me and said, "Don't worry." When Nick gives me that, I feel that I can go on...

Leni: Have you ever told him that directly?

Beth: I think I have.

Leni: Try telling him directly, because I noticed that you were addressing your remarks to the rest of us, rather than to Nick.

Beth: There is a big part of me that needs a father and needs everything a father can give: attention, love, affection.

I have needed to know that a father would soothe my crying and make me feel good again. You are giving that to
me and it really fills me up.

Leni: Did you know that?

Nick: I know I was trying. I didn't know I was successful.

The men's needs for sex and affection varied as much as the
women's. Some felt aroused by their partners' developing bodies. Others felt disinterested, timid or even repelled, expressing
their discomfort by withdrawing and becoming emotionally inaccessible or unconsciously spending more time away from home.
As their partners became more introverted and passive through
the months, the subsequent loss of attention sometimes became
equated with loss of love.

Nick: When Beth is so self-absorbed, I feel slighted by the
lack of attention, and I find myself becoming interested in
other women. I feel like a heel when I find myself flirting a
lot with other women.

In the first week, Dick wrote in his journal:

I feel apart from you, farther than we have been in months,
sometimes so far that it's as if I don't know you. I miss you.
You're sleeping a lot and lying around a lot. A feeling of a
friend rejected comes across me, but I don't reject you, too.
Perhaps I could massage you; I don't. I walk the dog for
you, buy specially requested food for you, cook for myself
and eat alone. Isn't that enough? Must I make love to you,
too? You are a beautiful woman and increasingly so. But are
you still the sexy woman? Seducing me and wanting me
between your legs like you did a month ago? Prove it. You
must come to me, not I to you.

Another father felt responsible for "ruining" his wife's body, as
it became more and more "distended." One admitted that his
image of his wife's breasts changed from a source of erotic pleasure to an image of two hanging milk dispensers. Such admis-

sions were not easy to make, but helped clear the way for better interactions. A few couples, however, had an active sex life until the last day, making love hours before labor started—despite their doctor's admonitions.

> **Nancy:** A great need came over me to be with John, but he was so immersed in his work that he didn't even seem to be aware of me. I started picking a fight with him, which was my sneaky way of getting him to pay attention to me. I started sobbing...I thought he didn't care. Of course, that wasn't true. He took me home and we made love. I knew instinctively that labor would not be far away after it. I think that was what my need was, to attend to myself pregnant, in the last hours of fullness, rather than let them slip away unacknowledged. At three A.M. I awoke John because I felt the birth waters oozing.

Dick was one of those who enjoyed each new development of his partner's changing body and felt aroused by her pregnant state

> I feel no less lust for her now than I ever did. In fact, I feel more attracted to her. It's simply one more aspect of the woman I love.

Beth felt beautiful and sexy, up until the last week:

> I'm doting on it—and my feeling of sexuality has been heightened. But in the past month (the ninth) I don't feel like having sex because I'm so puffy—orgasm is no longer down there, it feels like branches all around my body.

Ria wrote in her journal:

> I feel progressively less need for sexual intercourse as the pregnancy progresses, but increasing need for other physical contact with Eric—expressions of affection, concern, protection. More than sex.

Toward the end of pregnancy, it was a relief to be able to share problems about sex openly, knowing others in the group would understand.

> **Jean:** The lack of sexuality worried me. I didn't want sex, but I was worried that he didn't either. That was risky and scary. We got into a whole thing about who initiates sex. We couldn't even fit our bodies into each other. It was absurd—we had a few tragic episodes—I'd get a cramp— he'd freak and say, "It's moving"—it was hopeless.

> **Beth:** I know Nick felt he was hurting me or sometimes the baby and I felt awful about my body. It never worked by the end. And yet we really needed each other in that intimate way.

As developing bellies and the baby's movements confirmed the reality of the pregnancy, concern over impending motherhood became intertwined with thoughts of one's own mother. In the fourth and fifth months, women in the group began to relate to their mothers and the whole world of women in ways they hadn't for years. They were realizing that they were going to be mothers as well as daughters, just as their mothers were before them. Ria, whose mother lived in far distant Wisconsin, told us:

> I've been having a lot of feelings about my mother recently, angry feelings—wanting my mother to be more of what she isn't—more available on a deeper level. My mother is never available and I have been feeling a lot of resentment about that recently. Underneath is the fear that I will be that kind of mother, too. I want to be more giving and to be given to.

> **Elena:** Actually, I'm finding that my relationship with my mother isn't changed really, but there are subtle differences, especially in my attitude toward her. I feel more in need of her and I think of her frequently and feel more admiring of her now more than ever.
>   When I had morning sickness, there were a couple of times when I just thought, "I want my mother." I felt as sick

as I ever did when I was a kid and I want the total attention
my mother gave where every need was answered.

Anne was sitting next to her, crosslegged on the floor, supporting her back against Sam's legs. Leaning over to Elena, she
touched her hand and quipped:

I really know that feeling but I realized that I don't want *my*
mother. I want an archetypical one, the *perfect* mother,
don't you?

Women in the group reported that they spent lots of time
observing mothers and children in the park, on the bus, every-
where. They learned what they wanted and didn't want. They
also found they watched kids more than ever before. It was as if
their hearts opened up to all children as the pregnancy
advanced. They became archetypal mothers.

Men, too, began to think of their fathers sometimes wistfully,
sometimes with anger.

Don: I'm thinking a lot about the kind of father I want to
be. My dad wasn't home much. He was on the road a lot
for work. I don't want that. I want to be an important presence in my kid's life.

Dick: I can't imagine my father remembering my birth or
even my childhood. He was so remote. I really felt the loss
of his love. I was always trying to get his attention—sometimes pretty negatively.

John: I never was close to my father. He was always throw-
ing his power around. I never felt I was performing up to
snuff.

In their second trimester, women in the groups typically
moved from a concern for their relationship with their mothers,
to a preoccupation with their relationship to their partners. Most
of the women in the groups expressed an increasing need for
their husband's affection and concern. Often, they felt quite
dependent and needed reassurance, beyond what they them-

selves felt was acceptable or rational. By now the baby had "quickened in the womb," its activity a constant affirmation that it was alive and well; nevertheless, the women would often fret about whether things were progressing normally. Most of the men found these obsessive concerns difficult to deal with.

> **Peter:** I struggled to meet Jan's emotional needs, but often it got the best of me and I feel quite inadequate. After a while, I felt drained. No matter what I did, it was never enough. I began to feel hopeless. There was only so much attention I could give Jan—only so much hand-holding and reassurance. In a tribal society, there are more people around to help tend to the women.

> **Eric:** How many times can I assure Ria that the baby is not going to be a monster? I get very impatient.

They worried about what would happen in the future, after the baby arrived.

> **Elena:** I'm afraid it's going to be me and the baby together and Dick by himself out there. I get frightened and then he gets angry and then I get angry and I feel responsible, I want Dick to feel responsible, too. I want to know that I'm not in this alone.

They wanted their partner's involvement and sharing.

> **Anne:** I want you to feel the wonder of it just the way I feel the wonder of this unknown being who is soon to be known to us. I want you to know how it feels when the baby touches me inside...

> **Don:** With the most sympathetic interest and involvement, it is still something that is not happening to me—during the pregnancy, I'm a spectator.

> **Dick:** It's the most exceptional, and at the same time, rou- tine miracle in the world—a woman is just doing what she's

meant to do normally. Of course, I realize it's not routine to Elena, just collectively.

Don: Whatever you say about different societal attitudes over the centuries, giving birth is a power and a privilege— something that men are dwarfed by. I think it is a mysteri- ous thing—maybe that is why I take a step back from it, it is awesome and fearful.

But Amy wanted to be a *human*:

I don't want to be looked at like some goddess figure. I want your attention to be personal.

Men, too, were moving through a similar transformation as they became fathers to their children instead of sons to their fathers. Historically, men have been fearful of the transformative power of birth and in many cultures the birth process is per- ceived as a dangerous time. Some of that attitude carries over for both men and women now. In the groups, men and women alike harbored uncomfortable feelings about the messiness, bloodiness and potential danger of birth, remarking that they had read and heard it was a violent experience. One evening we spent time free-associating, starting with words such as blood, sex, mother, birth, breasts, pain, etc. Surprisingly negative atti- tudes and feelings were expressed. They recalled locker room stories and things their parents said.

Peter: When I think of birth, I can only think of all that stuff coming out...and of how bloody and dangerous it is.

Or women thought more specifically about the baby when they thought of birth.

I am worried about whether the baby will be normal. I was reading the *Time-Life* book on birth today, which is such an inhumane book, although an informational book, but saying things like—one of the most amazing things is that almost all of the systems in the baby have to start working right away...for instance, the lungs have never worked before. What if the lungs don't work, and the heart has only worked in a very simple way, and something new happens to the circulatory system when the baby's born. It changes, and what if it doesn't work?

Loss of control over one's body and over one's future became an imminent reality toward the end.

> **Jean:** The loss of control over what happens inside me is apparent. When I lie down to go to sleep. When I want to sleep, the baby starts to kick and I want to scream, "Stop!" I feel as if I am being taken over and things are moving much too fast. And that, quite possibly, I'm afraid to go to sleep for fear that I'll discover by morning that the baby has taken flight...or that I have died.

Thoughts of death were common toward the end among women and men. There was an intuitive sense that one's old self had to die, to be relinquished in order for the new parent self to born. But it was a struggle to accept the necessity of this transformation. One night, Ria confided:

> I have a fear of losing self—it's like a death—withering away and ecstasy are both a losing of self and I am fearful of both—of being carried away. Perhaps it is possible to go with the feelings no matter what they are.

> **Anne:** It's a point of vulnerability in your life, physical vulnerability. There's so much that's essential about life that's going on, but death is also present. I've become aware of both of them at the same time.

> **Eric:** When I think about the baby it makes me think about my mother's death last year, when we were only two months pregnant, about the continuum of family generations. She would have loved to be a grandmother. In fact, I'm just beginning to confront my own mortality.

Although we talked about problems that might arise during labor and delivery, and throughout the four months during which the group met, as the time of birth neared for some of the first couples, we focused more directly on specific questions and feelings. Fears were voiced about losing control, about one's ability to deal with pain, about trusting others to be there, giving support—fears about the unknown experience ahead.

And perhaps, underlying the unknown and the unpredictable aspects was the known—the unconscious "memory" for both parents of their own biological births, as Grof's and Sagan's theories suggest—colored by the fragments of recollections that parents and relatives hand down to us. These half-remembered memories and stories make us wary of reexperiencing the birth trauma once again, through the birth of our own children. There may also be an unconscious resistance to causing one's own baby pain during birth.

These fears can, indeed, affect the course of labor. Emotional anxiety can cause delays in contractions or create tension in uterine muscles, resulting in increased pain and prolongation of labor. As fear persists, the body responds by drawing blood away from the uterus toward organs of defense. As a result, the baby moving out of the womb and into the birth canal is deprived of the oxygenated blood on which its life depends, until it can start breathing on its own. Therefore it is of utmost importance to the well-being of both mother and child to give the kind of support that will dispel fear.

Dr. Grantly Dick Read contributed to "natural" childbirth in the 1940s with his book *Childbirth Without Fear*. It was the Read method that I practiced in New York City in 1949 for the birth of my first child. His ideas and methods are vitally important today. Although this may seem obvious now, it is essential to understand the biological consequences of anxiety, so that it can be eliminated as an inevitable aspect of childbearing. The best way to provide the needed support will be different for each mother and father.

In the early 1970s group members in the New York area had few alternatives to traditional hospital delivery. As with the majority of the population of the United States, cultural attitudes influenced their choice in favor of delivering in the hospital. Just like their parents, they followed the convention of the day. Decades before that, it was natural for their grandmothers to give birth at home in their own beds, attended by family physician or midwife, surrounded by their families. But, at this time, for these couples, the safety of the hospital environment, the modern technology of the delivery room and the care of the medical specialist were all crucial. So, all chose an obstetrician and planned to deliver in the hospital with which the doctor was affiliated. All couples attended a six-week "prepared" childbirth class that taught them breathing techniques to make labor easier. Most mothers looked forward to giving birth with a minimum of drugs. In the group, however, rather than concentrating on preparing for alternative ways of giving birth, we worked with the underlying feelings and emotions that *any* labor and delivery process would evoke.

Different concerns about labor and delivery arose for each couple. On one evening as pregnancies were coming to term, the recurrent issue of trust arose. This time it centered on the doubts Elena and Beth felt about their doctors.

> **Elena:** Since this is my first birth, I feel I have a right to go to Dr. F with my questions, even my simple questions, let alone the ones that I sense but can't articulate yet.
>
> You see, although I knew I could get answers to my questions out of a book, I wanted them from my doctor. I wanted his respect; I wanted him to know I could ask intelligent questions, that I knew what it was about. Because up until now, I've been sort of mute, which seems to be agreeable with him...I mean, he would say, "Do you have any questions?" and while saying that, be jumping out of the chair on the way to seeing the next person. So his attitude wasn't very conducive to an open exchange. It's as if I'm trying to say I want you to *see* me.
>
> **Beth:** I used to make a list of questions to ask my doctor, and, with my heart pounding for fear he'd refuse to answer, rush them all out, as he backed out the door. Often, about a

symptom, he'd say, "That's normal," leaving me totally dependent on his reassurance, without any information to help me be able to reassure myself.

We used another role-playing exercise in which Elena played the role of the doctor and others in the group played the roles of patient and husband. We acted out the office visit, asking all the questions that Elena was finding most difficult to articulate or even remember in the rushed exchange. As she took the role of her doctor, it allowed her to understand the doctor's position more clearly, and as her behavior was mirrored by someone else playing her part, it helped her to see her part in the interaction. We rehearsed the visit several times, finding that repetition brought self-confidence.

Many women in the group shared a fear that the doctor wouldn't be there with the emotional support they needed during labor. Hearing some of their friends' experiences had reinforced their anxiety and distrust. They also worried that they might lose courage at the last minute during labor and, despite their "training" and resolve to give birth without drugs, they might "chicken out."

One evening a casual discussion about the merits of home delivery resulted in an animated discussion involving trust of doctors and hospitals. Everyone interrupted each other in a rush to express themselves. It was a hot issue. We talked about control and about fear of the loss of control, and about taking responsibility for how we wanted things to happen. The men expressed confidence in the technological backup systems that would be available in the hospital environment. In contrast, many of the women not only were totally untrusting of this technology, but felt deeply threatened by the possibility of induced labor, fetal monitors, drugged delivery—all of it. Don had started out calmly and rationally:

I feel that the doctor is a professional: he knows what he's about, he's had a lot of training to do this and I trust him. I like to go to doctors.

But his partner, Amy, disagreed passionately:

> I resent doctors and hospitals. I feel as if I am putting myself in somebody else's hands. They don't tell you what they are doing and that includes my own doctor. I feel they are going to do something to me and not tell me....They are going to take it out of my hands at the hospital. That's been my experience every time I'm involved with a doctor.

Anne: I feel the same way really strongly.

Amy: I've been carrying this baby for nine months—it's been sleeping with me, been eating with me, living with me...By God, I've brought it this far, I can carry it the rest of the way.

Ria: Aren't you partly responsible for the way that happens? Can't you say to your doctor, "I don't want anything to happen to me without being specifically told"?

Anne: You can say that but some resident can come along and he's ready to induce and zap...,

Amy: You bet. The doctor gives me pat answers; he never explains anything no matter what I ask him. I see Don's role as fighting the doctor because I'm not going to have time to fight the doctor.

Eric: Can I ask you a question? Why in the world do you go to that doctor?

Amy: Because he's a good doctor.

Eric: Bullshit!

The evening ended with the issue unresolved, but the following week, we acted out a fantasy exercise in which we rehearsed the birth.

In another group, it was Ruth who was close to term, who began to worry about the feasibility of carrying out their plans.

> **Ruth:** Though I'm planning to have natural childbirth, I'm scared I might get scared at the end. I'll need my doctor's support then and where will he be? I want to be sure he'll be there as a guide and won't take it away from me at the last minute by making a decision for me, saying, "Oh, well, she's not doing too well, I'd better induce."

Like the others, Ruth was concerned about being pressured into accepting last-minute medical interventions, as had many of her friends.

At the next session, Ruth came to the workshop directly from her doctor's office, in a fury:

> I suddenly thought—who's in charge of all this? I am! Damn it. It's my body, my baby. It's hard to get into an accepting frame of mind when I ask the doctor questions and he answers, "This is the way we do it in the hospital...It is in your best interest." I come away believing for a while. I begin to agree with his reasoning. Yes, I really need an I.V. because if something goes wrong I might need an operation (does that become a self-fulfilling prophecy?), and I need an episiotomy because the tissue might rip and that would be terrible—I need a fetal monitor because the cord may strangle the baby or it may be stillborn but with this machine, they will save my baby. I begin to believe all these horror stories—it introduces all my worst fears and pretty soon I'm convinced. After all, I've gone to him assuming he knows. It's hard to say no, but damn, I'm yielding all my power to him—my mother instinct, the thing I trust inside. Suddenly I say to myself, wait a minute, I can't *trust* this doctor.

Ruth and her partner, Harvey, a psychiatrist at a large New York medical center, were concerned about planning the environment of their child's birth and were afraid that hospital rules and regulations would prevent them from creating it in their own way. Since Harvey was a doctor, he had first-hand knowledge of the system. Barring unforeseen complications, they wanted to design it their way. Ultimately they did—although the outcome was not what they had expected. In Chapter 5: The First Group Gives Birth, and in Chapter 6: Patterns and

Reflections: The Group Looks Back, their experience as well as that of others is described in relation to their long preparation in the group. In fact, there were three home births in the groups that I led. And these took place in New York City, not California. Two of those fathers were doctors, one father was an investment banker, his wife a foundation executive. All of the births proceeded without medical problems and each couple was very pleased with their choice.

Instructions for Emergency Childbirth

Perhaps the most important thing for the lay assistant to know is that labor and the delivery of a child are normal functions which nature always tends to complete satisfactorily....Underlying all basic principles is the realization that the performing of the delivery does not depend on the assistant, but on nature. To assist, he must have some idea of what nature is doing....Generally speaking, mechanical assistance is rarely needed, but psychological or emotional support to the mother is almost always in order....Such moral support is given to the mother not just because she is a fellow human being undergoing a trying experience, worthy as that reason is, but because calmness on her part and confidence in nature, in herself, and in her attendant make it possible for her to do her part of the job better. Giving birth, at its best, is something a mother does, not merely something which happens to her.

Police Training Manual of Chicago on Emergency Childbirth, A Manual,
Gregory J. White, M.D.

5

THE BIRTHING EXPERIENCE

It was such a miracle that first there was just
one person, and suddenly there were two.
—Sara, age 33, after the birth of Michael

Several weeks after the first workshop series had formally ended, we gathered once again to tell our stories. Three out of five babies had been born, and two couples had brought their infants to show them off to the group. More importantly, we wanted to share the details of the birth experiences before the intensity of the memories was lost. Of course, there had been the euphoric telephone calls immediately after the births to all of us as "extended family," but this evening of minute detail was an important follow-up. We were delighted to see each other.

Hearing this information had significant ramifications for the parents of the babies who had not yet been born. The exchanges that evening dramatically altered how some decided to shape the environment of their birth experience.

* * * *

Part of the ritual of becoming a mother is adding one's own history of giving birth to that of all the mothers who have given birth. It is not without meaning that thirty years later, a woman can tell her story in minute detail. Each mother is a central figure in the retelling of the mythic story of creation—the heroine's journey. It is akin to men telling their war stories—the hero's journey.

The relating of the birth story can become unexpectedly poetic, as in the following journal entry from Sara:

> When the time came to push, a surge went rippling through my body and soul demanding that I bear down so that I could push life into the world like all the other women before me who have chosen to be passages to life.
>
> Within seconds of his head crowning, his body slipped out of mine, an ooze and a swish that felt glorious and was too quickly gone. Like seeing the morning sunrise, there are no words to speak my heart at this moment. I am in awe. I ache with joy.

As the women talked, I was aware of a fascinating change in the group's interactions. This change was striking to me: After so many months of intimacy, couples who had given birth were now absorbed in the demands of parenthood. These concerns had catapulted them beyond the reach of their still-pregnant friends. The latter were still coping with some of their fears about the unknown and unpredictable transition that lay ahead of them. There was an unacknowledgable, subtle emotional distance between the two groups—those who had crossed the bridge into the future and those who waited to do so. And the tiny members of the group, who had been present but not seen before, became an irresistible focus of attention, try as we might to cling to the old group patterns. Gradually, the group molded itself to include these wonderful new distractions. It was moving to see mothers who had worried so about their competence now caring for their babies as if they had been doing so forever.

Of the three births, two were complicated hospital deliveries that had proved to be quite traumatic for the whole family.

Even after attending a support group such as ours, and having the advantage of more preparation that usual, parents had remained powerless to carry out their plans. It was clear that the medical system, even in these different "excellent" hospitals of the parents' choice, was not responsive to the essence and nature of the birth event. This revelation affected one still-expectant couple so strongly that they began making plans for a home delivery at a friend's house near their hospital. Ria and Eric, whose delivery was less stressful, were able to carry out their personal plans more successfully.

AMY AND DON

Amy and Don's experience of labor and delivery was, they believed, not what they had expected—or wanted—at all.

> It's amazing. It was nothing like anything I was prepared for beforehand. I remember feeling that with all my reading and all of my exercise and our work together here, I was going to have a snap of a time. Never did I consider that it would be as it was.

First of all, Amy's doctor was on vacation, so his partner took over. He sent her to the hospital when she was dilated three centimeters and in the course of the next eight hours, her labor moved along very slowly; she dilated only one more centimeter. Nurses and interns came and went as day staff were replaced by night staff.

> As soon as I became comfortable with one, he or she turned into another. The doctor came in and told me he could speed up my labor by giving me Pitocin. I knew that meant it would be much more painful and they would have to give me painkilling drugs to offset the pain. I was not prepared for that. Never had I considered that I would take any kind of anesthesia because of its effect on the baby. When I asked him what was happening, he told me he didn't know but it must be something in my midbrain. I didn't know what happened in my midbrain, but I figured that it was something psychological. I figured I wasn't natural enough to have natural childbirth. I got very upset and even more tense. He never even explained to me what happens in your midbrain.

The doctor and nurses put pressure on Amy to agree to having an epidural (spinal anesthetic). Don was enlisted to convince her, too. They told her if she had an epidural and used Pitocin, she would have the baby in three hours; otherwise her labor might continue in the same slow, ineffective way for twelve hours.

> **Amy:** I didn't know what to do as they kept saying, "It's up to you. If I were you, I'd want to get it over with."

Reluctantly, feeling like a failure, she agreed.

As Amy talked that evening, I remembered something she'd said during an earlier workshop session. She had expressed her anxiety about submitting to the medical system, since a previous experience in the hospital for a small operation had been a bad one, in which they never told her what they were doing.

> When they gave me the spinal, they hit a nerve. I was so scared. I said, "Get away from me. Don't touch me. I'll do this birth myself." "O.K.," they said, "if that's the way you feel," and they took out everything and walked out. The doctor got mad at me and wouldn't talk to me. One thing led to another. Meanwhile, I was in a lot of pain. Don was pressuring me to get them back in to administer the spinal again. Hours passed, no further dilation, no progress, nothing. I felt like a failure. Was I blocking the baby? Then the contractions started again and they were so painful that I soon took the Demerol they offered. Afterward, the doctor walked in, donned rubber gloves, did a vaginal exam, checked the chart and walked out without saying a word. After several such visits, Don followed him out of the room and insisted on knowing what was the matter. I finally gave in and asked for the epidural. We went through the whole performance again. When the anesthesiologist returned to give me the epidural this time, it worked. They numbed me. We went to the delivery room and I kept saying, "Should I push now?" "Don't bother," was the doctor's curt answer. Meanwhile, when the doctor left the room, the nurse was guiding me and encouraging me to push and she kept telling me how well I was doing. After a short while, the

doctor reappeared, saw me pushing and said, "You can push till doomsday. Nothing will happen." He never explained why. Then, without saying a word to me, he took out forceps and started to insert them. I didn't know what was happening. A resident came in and the doctor started to lecture him that the baby was turned wrong. In the mirror above me, I watched him pull on my baby's head with the forceps. It was awful. I felt so sad for my baby, and I was worried about its tiny, soft head, as the doctor tugged on it. The baby, in fact, was born with bruises on its head.

After the birth, the anesthesiologist said to Don and me, "Only one doctor in a thousand could have performed such a feat. Other doctors would have performed a caesarean." Maybe that's true, but I'm not sure. I felt the men and women attendants at the hospital were so different; the men acted like medical knowledge was a private cache. I ended up feeling helpless.

Ria and Eric were the next to report that night.

RIA AND ERIC

When labor started for Ria, she and Eric stayed at home as long as possible, since she was determined not to spend unnecessary hours in the hospital. Arriving at the hospital, in active labor, she had to undergo routine hospital procedures: enema, intravenous drip, pubic shave. After examination by a resident, she was put to bed. At that point, her labor, too, stopped cold just as Amy's had, and they had hours of waiting without further dilation. They provided comfort for themselves by bringing some pieces of their home environment with them: a favorite quilt, some poetry, music, cards and most important, a trusted friend and Lamaze teacher to be labor coach. Somehow, the friend was able to breeze through the labor room doors with them and the three of them were ensconced there, waiting it out. Although their doctor had been told that their labor coach was coming along and was in favor of it, he hadn't cleared her presence with the hospital authorities. Consequently, he spent many of the hours during the labor battling with the power structure to allow her to remain.

> **Ria:** Fathers were accepted in the labor and delivery rooms, but a third undefined person wasn't normal, so it was a big hassle. The doctor wanted to win this political battle so that others in the future would not have the same problem.

Proud that their doctor was eager to confront the system, they nevertheless felt abandoned during his absence as he did battle, acting as guardian of the gate instead of wise counselor-comforter during most of the labor. By the time Ria was on the delivery table, he returned and their chosen team was reunited to give her the emotional support she needed during the birth.

> **Ria:** All of us were crying for joy as the baby emerged. I was really high, even through the heavy dose of Demerol I had taken. It ended up just fine. No epidural, just Demerol. Demerol was O.K. With anything else, I wouldn't have been able to push effectively. My baby hadn't turned in the pelvis either, as Amy's hadn't, and if I hadn't been able to push, the doctor would have had to use forceps. It would have been a far more complicated delivery. As it was, it was comparatively easy, so I'm convinced that there are things that are done in the way birth is managed that interfere with what we women do naturally.

ANNE AND SAM

The workshop sessions were over several months before Sam and Anne's baby was due. They had joined very early in their pregnancy. After hearing the troubling stories of their friends' hospital deliveries, they opted for a home birth. Even though their choice carried its own anxieties, they felt as though it would allow them more control over how their baby began its life.

Fortunately for them, their obstetrician, an older woman renowned in her field, agreed to deliver their baby at the apartment of close friends. Interestingly, their obstetrician was the partner of mine who had delivered my third child decades before. The friends, a couple who were both doctors, lived a

few blocks from their physician's hospital. They felt very fortunate to be able to make these arrangements.

Anne's labor was prolonged. At one point, contractions
recurred ten minutes apart for thirty-six hours. Then they
petered out, like Amy's.

> **Anne:** I meditated on what was going on with me, trying to
> sense myself. I decided it was up to me. No one could do it
> for me or to me. I never felt anything was wrong, just slow.
> Interestingly, during those three days of labor, I never expe-
> rienced any of the fears I had discussed in the group, fear
> of death or anything else. Maybe I had worked them
> through.

> **Leni:** Were you feeling comfortable with the Lamaze
> breathing exercises: Was the panting helpful?

> **Anne:** Yes, that became very automatic. I didn't even stop
> to calculate. I thought for a while that we'd have to figure
> out which kind of breathing I should be doing, depending
> on how long the contractions were. I thought it was going
> to be a big head trip, but somehow, I used the breathing as
> I felt I needed it. I just came out. I didn't bother with focus-
> ing on a certain point of whatever; it just became a tool that
> was just part of me, and it worked very well.
>
> At one point, after all those hours, the doctor thought it
> (the baby) was in posterior position, "Now I know why
> you've been putzing around for these two days," she said.
> "That's very common with posteriors."
>
> I had this back pain, so I really wanted somebody there
> pushing on my back, and we tried the different positions
> Lamaze recommends for the back. Our childbirth educator
> had recommended that we take the course to prepare for
> breathing during labor. That was helpful. I still wanted
> everyone's interaction.
>
> Then I went into transition labor, although I wasn't really
> conscious of it except that my breathing started to be differ-
> ent. That was very painful, as it turned out. I think it was
> because of the posterior thing. A few times toward the end
> of the transition when the pain was really bad, I was having
> trouble staying on top of it.

After that, she examined me and said, "You're fully dilated." At that point, she and Sue were into their technical
thing...I mean, the doctor had instruments and things, I
guess an umbilical clamp or whatever. I had no desire to
master what they were doing. I had such respect and trust
for the two of them, that I could let them do their own
thing. It is such a relief not to have to think, "Oh my God—
they are down at the foot of the bed collaborating, thinking
up something to do to me." It was just another example of
how being at home was so fantastic. I was able to give up
my whole compulsion about being part of *all* the decisions
that physicians make. I felt I could really trust them, let
them do their thing and take care of myself. Throughout all
of this time, though, we were working together. I really
very much had this sense, and I keep describing the birth as
the six of us doing it.

The interaction was so smooth and so alive and it was
really terrific. I just never would have gotten through this at
all on my own. I never would have. I would have been too
discouraged and gone to the hospital and done the Pitocin
thing. But here at home, everybody was leaving it to me.
Nobody was pushing any of their thing on me—including
the physician—leaving it to me, all the way through.

Leni: It was just what you wanted. I remember you had
said earlier, "I don't want people interfering with me. I want
Sam there to protect me and to help make sure that what I
want, I can be clear about. And if I'm not clear, I want protection so I can have time to become clear and not be
messed with."

Anne: The doctor got me into incredibly active pushing.
Then she withdrew and sat on the end of the bed. Sam and
Sue came up and the three of us were pushing. It was so
different from our practice sessions with Lamaze. In this situation, the three of us were a whole unit of energy. In
between contractions, too, I was hanging onto hands—one
on each side. The energy coming through the hands was
really something. I just lay back and absorbed the flowing
energy between contractions and then I was ready to do
another.

Sam: I got to see the results of different things that we tried. I had both of my hands behind her back supporting her and I noticed after the second push that there was no progress. When I pushed with her, she pushed back very hard...it was all I could do to support her strength in pushing.

And I could see, I could look right down between her legs and see the baby's head push out and come back each time.

Anne: Sue would say, "I can see, it's a quarter." Then she'd say, "It's fifty cents. You've got to make it an orange." I was tuned into just everything around me and my body, too. Incredible. I just—I had partly, from video tape and a couple of films that I saw of birth, had this whole picture—I was seeing it in my head. My eyes were absolutely shut during the whole pushing thing, but I was seeing an entire scene. I knew what it looked like. Really, really marvelous. Also from inside, I was absolutely acutely aware of every sensation. For instance, between contractions, as the baby would move back deeper into the birth canal I remembered similar feelings to how he would move when he was in the womb, when he would shift his body around. I can't tell you how acute my sensations were—I was totally into that part of me, completely.

I could feel the doctor rotating his head because he had been posterior.

We decided the next pushing series would bring the baby out. I asked her whether I should be holding back after the head comes out. She said, "Yes, I'll tell you when to stop pushing." When the head came out, she said, "O.K., hold it." I was panting. I was soaking wet.

The doctor put her finger in and just turned him with a flip, pulled his head around the right way and he came out.

Sam: It was exciting. I could see the head crowning. It would appear and then disappear. What seemed to help the baby at that point, was a great deal of physical support of Anne's back. I tried to give her something strong to lean against by placing my arms and chest under her back. The force of the contractions was powerful. I had a tennis elbow

for three weeks afterward, but more important than my discomfort was my feeling that I helped my baby to get born. I
had a real sense of participation.

He was crying and he wasn't even out yet, and then all
of a sudden he was out, and he was sitting there—this glis-
tening light, and he *still* was crying. When he came out, he
was absolutely pink.

After the birth, the doctor handed me the scissors and
asked me to cut the cord. It was translucent and beautiful,
with the consistency of rubber hose. I cut it slowly.

Our pediatrician friend who attended us checked our son
out immediately, and after Anne held him and fell asleep
herself Mark fell asleep in the cradle. A few hours later, he
woke up and Anne was resting. I picked him up and held
him in my arms as I watched the ball game. I knew he was
mine. No question about that. I didn't have to see him
through the window.

RUTH AND HARVEY

In a subsequent group, it was the first rather than the last couple
to give birth who once again felt pressed into choosing a home
delivery. Over several sessions, we had worked through various
exercises as had the former group: a visit to the doctor and a
rehearsal of the birth. The next week, Ruth and Harvey went for
their appointed visit to the obstetrician armed with very specific
questions. Since Harvey was a physician himself, there was
added weight in his presence. They confronted the doctor with
questions about routine procedures. He answered that he did
require an I.V. during labor so that in case there was need for
emergency medication it would be right there. Yes, he would
use a fetal monitor if necessary. In fact, he told them that just
the other night a baby of one of his patients would have been
stillborn if he had not used the monitor. When asked about an
episiotomy, he said he'd wait and see, but for the first birth it's
usually a routine procedure!

Ruth: I kept thinking, I sure hope he's patient. He gave
very reasonable medical answers to all our questions and

we kind of "yes"-ed along until we got home and started thinking it through. I began to realize that he might not even be at my birth; it might be one of his two associates. That threw me. I didn't want that at all. Sure, I had already met them. Quick introductions. In two minutes it was over. I never had the chance to talk with them. I told him I really wanted *him* to deliver the child, that I felt close to him, but he told me he couldn't promise that. However, he had arranged it so that he would be the one that I would see for my next two appointments before the due date. When it came right down to making the appointments, he was all booked up for the first and second times and I had to see the other doctors anyway. That did it! We began to plan for a home delivery. We decided we would plan to give birth at home, if the baby was in a normal position.

Since Harvey worked in a large city hospital, he felt confident that he would be able to find a physician or midwife to attend them at home. It turned out to be an almost impossible task. Their fruitless search surprised us all. Finally, they learned that the nurse who was the head of the intensive care unit at Harvey's hospital had been a midwife for many years in her native Jamaica, and she agreed to come. Ruth and Harvey were pleased at their good fortune.

Having decided to deliver at home, they invited the group members to be present, along with Ruth's parents, Harvey's son from a former marriage and several close friends.

A week later, at four p.m., Harvey called and asked me to come as soon as I could. "Ruth's in labor!"

The group arrived from all over, at different intervals, most coming directly from work. My coleader, Tom, flew in from a medical meeting in Boston. Ruth's labor started in earnest at about five o'clock. The emotional energy in the room was extraordinary.

Ruth looked beautiful. She sat on the bed with her legs folded under her, rocking rhythmically through each contraction, her head and body rolling, her eyes closed, the long loose white caftan she was wearing yielding to the shape of her full breasts and moon belly.

At first, as we gathered around Ruth, there was tentativeness in each of us in such an unfamiliar circumstance. That soon passed as we became absorbed in the drama and power of the event in which we were participating. Each of us began to sense when and how to comfort Ruth by massaging or stroking her between contractions, with the midwife's sensitive guidance. Being with a couple during birth is a sacred form of sharing and each of us was conscious of that.

At eleven P.M., after six hours of intense labor, Aaron was born. At that moment, I felt we all touched eternity. It was impossible to be silent.

Awe, wonder, ecstasy, relief, joy and love mingled in a tender swelling fugue of murmuring sound. The actual words mattered not at all. The midwife placed the baby at Ruth's breast and Harvey lay down beside them on the big bed. When the cord stopped pulsating, Harvey cut it and gently immersed his new-born son in the warm bath that had been readied. Aaron was quietly alert, splashing gently, following our movements and looking attentively at each of us in the room. Soon after, Ruth delivered the placenta. Harvey wrapped the baby in a towel and, with no need for words, the room emptied, each of us sensing their need to be alone.

A week later, the words flowed freely:

> **Ruth:** It certainly hurt a lot, especially during the last ten contractions or so, but it had its rhythm, its compelling force. There was just no way I could stop, no turning back. I just had to do it to keep moving with it...I remember say-ing in one of our sessions, "I wonder what makes the baby come out? What is that thing?" Now, I know. I read all those books about the physical part and the medical part and the breathing techniques and what to do with herbs and all of it. When it came right down to it, it was my heart that gave birth to the baby. It wasn't my breathing, it wasn't the con-trol of the breath, panting and all, it was heart that was so strong in that room.
>
> Having the whole group there with me was tremendous. You know, as everyone gathered round me for those hours, I never really knew whose hands were stroking me; it didn't

matter; it was a continuous stream of love and reinforcement. I just remember looking up at one point and seeing Ellen standing opposite me, her pregnant belly quivering, her eyes filled with tears. Our eyes met for what seemed like an eternity.

The responses from others present at the birth were colored by the unique needs and personal expectations that each brought to an intense experience like this one.

Ellen, the pregnant woman, and Tom, the coleader-doctor, both expressed their reactions in some detail.

Ellen later said that being there was incredible for her:

> I remember wondering about all my anxieties, about all the questions that I thought I would be asking, like, "Is the baby strangling or is it breathing? Is the cord around its neck?" It all sort of went out the window when I saw the dark spot get bigger and bigger and then it came out. I kept thinking it's born and yet nothing official's happening. No people running around, no equipment, no metal, no white things. Just a warm intimate scene. All the while, I knew that it is not going to be this particular way for me. One part of me was thinking, on the other hand, I'll feel safe and I'll feel that everything is going to be all right there in the hospital. I know I can't muster that feeling up for myself at home the way Harvey and Ruth have, but can it be the kind of celebration it was for them in the hospital environment? While watching Ruth give birth, a huge burden of fear dropped off me. It just fell away. Ruth was deeply absorbed. I knew she was O.K. The midwife was "ironing" the perineum, stretching it and waiting patiently for Aaron to emerge in his own time.
>
> It was really incredible. I felt death there as life was beginning. It was awesome, not frightening, not morbid, just awesome and it was O.K. To feel death was as miraculous as to feel life. Not the death of a person, just those absolutes, life and death, side by side, a brush with eternity. There was a moment when he was half in Ruth's body and half out, when his face was so blue and the force of him was so enormous...I had a feeling that he was determining

whether he was going to do it or not, whether he was going to go the rest of the way. There was a split second when time was eternal...then it was like fast motion when it was as if the baby decided he was going to come out.

Tom, as a doctor, had concerns that were somewhat different from Ellen's. He reflected later:

There was so much life energy in the room—birth energy— so much beauty—it was powerful. We must be afraid of it in our culture, because we certainly suppress it. Instead, our culture breeds fear into us about the birth process and we act out of it. I was so aware of my medical responses, that God forbid, because she was straining and it was taking a long time—or it seemed like a long time—something was going to go wrong and I would have to do something about it. In fact, everything was working just fine; Ruth was working, the baby was working, the midwife was working. It was that natural force that my medical conditioning was prepared to turn off. I realized how we turn it off deliberately, expensively, completely. Really, it's just like that. As doctors, we are not trained to respond to good; we are trained to respond to bad and no amount of reality testing seems to convince us that bad things don't happen as often as good things. We're trained that if we do it wrong, we're going to get into trouble. If a doctor has a setback, he'll take it out on a thousand patients after that. Being at Aaron's birth was so important for me as a physician. It made me aware and appreciative of the self-regulation aspects of the life process. I realize now why people get so angry about home delivery. They are overwhelmed by the awesome quality of the life force. Of course, there are dangers. Some babies do have trouble breathing. There can be hemorrhaging, and we need to be prepared for that; and even then, sometimes babies die! We must be willing to accept death as part of life. That's the ultimate risk. The risk was present in that room for each of us. It's the end as well as the beginning. It's as if the process is in reverse. I've watched people die, watched the letting go process, letting the breath out. For Aaron, it was the way it sounds in reverse, a gentle beginning sound—"Ahhh," for a few seconds, not long—then taking hold.

In addition to my personal memories of the group sessions and the births, I had hours of videotape records of our sessions. My next task, as part of my doctoral thesis project, was to create an hour-long documentary that might eventually be used as part of a prenatal counseling support system by health professionals. I had to edit twenty-six hours down to two one-half hour tapes. It was a monumental job, but I found the tapes to be very exciting and dramatic, in the sense that reviewing the material over a short time period highlighted certain patterns I hadn't noticed before. In the course of analyzing and editing the tapes, it was necessary to go over the tapes again and again. The words bounced around in my head. Over and over again, the same sentences were repeated until they were imprinted on my memory.

I was struck by the fact that each couple, early in the pregnancy, had virtually predicted the way in which labor and delivery would happen for them. They said it in many different ways at separate intervals, often unrelated to speculations about labor and delivery. In the final tape, I placed the earlier and later statements in flashback sequence—the effect was startling. This surprising observation raised the whole question of the role of self-fulfilling prophecies in affecting what happens to us. Do we decide how some events in our life will proceed and then act out these prophecies? The birth experiences of Amy and Don and Ruth and Harvey might be seen as examples of this intriguing possibility.

My insights into the nature of the individual couples' birth experiences came directly out of working closely together as a support group for so many months. I believe not only that such groups are essential, but that they are not enough. It is necessary for us to design an environment for childbearing that integrates all aspects of birth into people's life experience, the physiological, emotional, spiritual, medical. Then this passage, this crucial event, can be viewed as part of the weave of the human tapestry, a new design, and not a rent or a tear in what should be continuous and smooth.

As a result of my work with these warm, caring couples, it became clear to me that the quality of the emotional intimacy between the people involved was perhaps the most important element influencing the environment of pregnancy and birth.

Even the proponents of "natural" or "prepared" childbirth sometimes seem so intent on the virtues of their various methods that the deep emotional quality of the experience of birth is overlooked, as if that part will take care of itself. The kind of intimacy that is needed during labor and delivery doesn't spring full blown suddenly as contractions begin. The capacity for holding each other tenderly requires slow and tender nurturing, that comes from the heart. During times of emotional stress, we discover only what has been there all the time. The crisis of this rite of passage simply amplifies the emotions already present. It seems to me that our fears and anxieties are only fulfilled if we don't let go, can't surrender. If we can loosen the emotional knots beforehand, the necessary physiological surrender will come more easily.

Preparation for the complex emotional and physical demands of childbirth should begin long before the actual event. We have much to learn. Telling our stories—and listening—is a beginning.

6

PATTERNS, RECOLLECTIONS, REFLECTIONS

Awareness doesn't cause *change—awareness* is *change*
—Dick

Because the workshops were designed as creative psychological explorations rather than scientific experiments, it is neither possible nor desirable to evaluate them in scientific terms. Nor have I made any attempt to draw rigorous conclusions from the responses of the many people who met with me over the years. What I offer here is a report on our work as carried out this far—one model in a development process, reflecting my particular intuitive psychological and environmental focus on family development during a significant normal life transition. Other groups would undoubtedly reflect their particular personalities and specific needs. In Chapter 7, I suggest some ways to start and structure groups—with or without leaders, small or large, etc.—that may be useful in helping you design the group that is best for you.

After each workshop series came to an end, I asked group members to evaluate their experience. Shortly after each birth, I personally visited as many couples as I could and we discussed their reactions to participation in the group and their feelings about the birth of their child. Their responses helped me to redesign the structure of future groups to make the process more effective.

When I decided to make this material available in a book, I knew I wanted more specific reactions and evaluations of the group process by the people who had been most involved.

Thus, six years later, I found myself trying to contact as many parents as I could locate. Some were still close enough to visit in person, others I interviewed on the phone. It was typical of our mobile American culture that parents had moved to various parts of the country: California, Pennsylvania, Maryland, Vermont, and Washington State. Some I had lost track of entirely. However, untypical of contemporary United States, among the fifteen families I contacted, only one couple was divorced. This news was extremely gratifying to me, and I hoped—although I could not assume—that their stability as families was related to the emotional support they had received during the group sessions; and the opportunity to work through some of their problems at a crucial period in their lives.

During this period it became necessary for me to return to New York from my home in Northern California. Before my trip east, where some of the couples from the original groups still lived, I sent out a questionnaire in order to stir up memories of the group experience. I was aware of how much my own life had changed in the intervening six years, and knew the parents would need a little time to recapture the emotional climate of that pregnant year. I also wanted to stimulate thinking about the broader ramifications and possible applications of what we had learned.

In the following section, I present their answers and some of my reflections on their replies. I hope this material provides useful insights, not only into the nature of the workshops, but into the pregnant year itself. These couples spent a tremendous amount of time and energy becoming aware of their changing needs before and after the birth of their children, and their present feelings about themselves and their children reflect their increased sensitivity to many issues, a sensitivity and concern that were definitely fostered by their participation in the group sessions.

RIA AND ERIC

After Ria finished her nursing degree, she spent weekdays in New York completing midwifery training while Eric worked full-time at his job teaching in Massachusetts, where they lived. He has been the major caretaker of their two children (Kathy and Neil). They have since moved to the midwest, where Ria will be a midwife in a large urban hospital. Eric is now the director of a national program for young mothers and fathers that teaches early parenting.

After Kathy's birth, Ria was one of the few who had responded to the original questionnaire:

> The group experience was very important to us. It gave us the opportunity to think out loud about how we wanted Kathy's birth to happen. As we listened to the others, our ideas took form, and ultimately we were able to affect our hospital experience to some degree...not enough, but it was something. Our doctor was affected, too. We became far better clients, were able to ask far more specific questions and were able to talk to him about our feelings, since they were brought to a conscious level. We also affected the hospital. I nursed Kathy on the delivery table...a first in that hospital. They won't forget us in a hurry. I hope that softened the way for others.
>
> We both find the question, "What did you get out of the group?" so difficult to answer...what happened to us was such a complex experience, which we've not fully analyzed. Summarizing seems almost impossible.
>
> I had become interested in the psychology of pregnancy through my schoolwork, and also felt there were issues to be dealt with by the pregnant couple, which could be handled well in a group. I still had a rather vague sense that Eric and I were not enjoying our pregnancy as much as we might.
>
> For years I had been told by a gynecologist that I would probably not be able to conceive without intervention or medication or surgery, so I was immensely pleased to find myself pregnant. But, as the pregnancy was not planned, and began just as Eric's mother was dying, and since he was

reluctant to have a baby until I finished nursing school, I was worried about how things would work out for us as a couple.

I didn't know what I felt should be happening, but so much of the time I felt the pregnancy was just within me...rather than within us...and that was a lonely feeling, a frightening one. I didn't know what was wrong, but felt that something definitely was not right, and so looked to the group, as a chance for Eric and me to be more fully together.

As I look back, I realize how little I knew of what was missing. It was only through the group, which released us to fulfill so much more of our potential for sharing, that Eric and I learned how far apart we had been.

What happened to me in the group was, I think, a general sort of release. Eric and I began to talk more and more, and to work together in planning for the birth and child care. The feelings I'd had inside me all along (positive and negative) found their ways into words, and in sharing with others, I discovered new ideas and feelings about pregnancy and birth, and children and parenting. It was terribly exciting, and a strengthening experience for me. My loneliness subsided a good deal . . . I-we became more alive and open to pregnancy, with its joys and deepest fears.

And yet we didn't really deal with the issue of Eric's anger about the unplanned pregnancy, nor with the question of whether I was to blame for that event. We must have talked all around it without ever looking at this issue straight on. And it has continued to be a source of tension and mistrust in our relationship, which we are just now beginning to try to explore.

I had no idea that Eric was as angry as he was about the unplanned baby, nor that he felt I'd tricked him into pregnancy. I wished that I had been able to open up about it in the group instead of holding back, when I had the opportunity.

Six years after Kathy's birth, Ria responded in her usual thoughtful detail to my second questionnaire:

We *have* recommended group experiences to people going through various pregnancies—that is, we've often talked about our group and the value it had for us, and encouraged people to put together their own support groups, especially if childbirth education classes aren't meeting their needs. The fact is that such groups are not usually available, and they need to be started. My current idea is that once I get settled in a job as a staff midwife, Eric and I can teach childbirth classes together and create a group experience along the lines of the group we had with you. A group that deals with the whole experience of being pregnant and giving birth, becoming a family. I know that we needed your group (our group) quite apart from our preparation for childbirth series, and there was more work to do than could be fit in around the relaxation exercises, etc.—but as a midwife, I really don't see how one can do the one without the other...

I think a similar group would have been great for our pregnancy with our second child. The openness was there again, some of the same issues were asking to be dealt with, and there were certainly as many changes to be coped with as the first time around—different ones, but as many. It's really a matter of taking advantage of a unique time for growth as individuals and as a couple—as a family, too... We were so concerned about Kathy's sharing in Neil's birth, and as I will probably tell you somewhere down the line, it was surprising to find how little we had prepared *ourselves* for the change in her life.

Yes, indeed, if we were pregnant again, we would both want a group.

I would recommend that a group use your lovely audio tape *The Child Within* as an aid to their group.

The most difficult aspect of my first pregnancy was dealing with the relationship between Eric and me. We became pregnant with a lot going against us, I think: unplanned pregnancy; me in school and Eric's mother terminally ill with leukemia (she died when I was two months pregnant).

The list could probably go on but this is enough! At any rate, much of this was just simmering away in each of us, not being talked about very much, not being dealt with in any productive way, and giving rise to a lot of anger which came out in other ways, creating a lot more tension between us.

I remember worrying because Eric never brought up the subject of the pregnancy, never wanted to touch my belly. I was basically pleased to be pregnant (though not without a lot of mixed feelings). I remember Lucy Ann's suggesting the group, and then suggesting it myself to Eric. My memory is that he was reluctant at first but agreed to do it. That was when we began to be pregnant *together*. We had the one night a week which we saved for ourselves, for the pregnancy and the baby and trying to come to grips with what was happening to us.

It was so incredibly important that we had the baby together. I look back on the experience and can see all kinds of problems which had to be worked out later on, but we made progress then, and I think if we hadn't we might well not have gotten through the even harder (in some ways) times ahead for us as a couple.

The easiest and most joyful aspect of the pregnancy was the physical experience of carrying a child, and then the actual childbirth. And then, I think, *the* most joyful aspect of the entire process was falling in love with Kathy, and with ourselves as a family—but that has been for us a gradual process, a growth into more excitement and joy. It certainly didn't happen immediately when she was born, although we were both very thoroughly engrossed in her from the beginning. I found the hospitalization lonely, uncomfortable emotionally and sometimes physically, too, full of annoying routines—but I also have a very special feeling about that time: the smell of Vaseline, the Jamaican voices, my baby being wheeled in during the night to be nursed and then just curled up on my bare chest afterwards to sleep; my body going through all those enormous changes, all normal and purposeful and deeply exciting to me.

Eric: We came into the group after being "recruited" by a friend. We didn't know much about what the group would involve, but expected an expansion of the Lamaze material. In retrospect, for me Lamaze appears to need a great deal of expansion, and the group showed clearly how many issues are not explored in the skill-oriented Lamaze ses-

sions. Lamaze feeds right into the technology of the hospital—an approach not broad enough to encourage more creative dealing with the complex questions involved in
childbearing.

Earlier, I felt tricked into having a baby...Ria had wanted
it, not me...When the group began, I was having a hard
time thinking about the baby at all or about myself as a
father. I'd considered our pregnancy helpful not for me but
for my father, giving him a "life" focus after my mother's
recent death. But that wasn't me. One of the major impacts
of the group on me was that it forced me to think of myself
as a father and permitted me to think about my fathering
fantasies...In the course of the workshop, I moved from not
having thought much about the baby at all to saying that I
wanted a major part of the responsibility for childcare after
the birth. Actually, the group experience facilitated expression of my ideas about involvement. They were part of me,
I know, but might never have been expressible or capable
of development unless I had them shared with others.

ELENA AND DICK

Elena is a social worker with a poetic bent. After the birth of
their first daughter, Becky, she started to do some personal writing, some of which has since been published. Dick is an architect who works for a large design firm. They are still living in
New York.

Elena and Dick's new baby daughter, Ellie, was three months
old when I visited them in New York some years later. It was
their second daughter.

Elena: I think I'm quite different with this baby, and that
makes her different. I guess I trusted my feelings more this
time. I also feel we're more mature.

Dick: It's true. We didn't talk about it a lot this time, but I
was more aware of your feelings. However, I didn't talk
about my feelings this time. Actually, you did. Do we use
each other in this way? Yes, I think that old pattern still
holds. If you worry, then I don't have to and vice versa...

We divide up the issues of concern and collude together—when you worry, I have to be the caretaker.

Elena: We were very involved without our own parents during the first time…psychologically. I really wanted my mother around that first pregnancy, I remember. She came but stayed with her sister. Maybe I should have been more explicit about asking her to stay with me. Then she fell down on the way over to see me and arrived bleeding, needing my help just when I needed her! Her solution was to call up her twin sister and ask her to come instead. Even though she didn't do those nice motherly things like get tea, I wanted her. Then it was amazing…She said, "I know how scared you are," and that opened up a lot. Since she was not giving me what I needed, I had to get it somewhere else.

But I have trouble asking people for help. In my childhood, I recall my mother saying, "Neither a borrower nor a lender be." I realized during this pregnancy that I was basically alone. At the same time, I also knew that I could get what I needed if I was grown up about handling it. I realized that was what maturity was about. Maturity is learning that you can make your own choices.

I never thought of it as a therapy group, though I suppose it was. I think when you call it a support group, it's much less threatening. You're very vulnerable when you're pregnant and getting "therapized" is a scary thought, though one may need exactly that. If you call it a support group, then you can explore just what a support group is.

You know, you need a lot of mothering during pregnancy. The father needs it, too. Dick let his feelings out more than most men but he got neglected by me. In the group, men got paid attention to. Did you ever consider that we think it's terrific if a pregnant woman's mother comes to take care of her daughter and makes it easier, especially during and after the birth, but no man's mother rushes over to take care of her son! He needs a lot, too. In fact, the final straw may be that the mother-in-law rushes over to take care of her daughter-in-law.

Dick: It's true this time I felt even more excluded. Last time, I wanted to run away. Maybe this time there was a letdown because the group was not there. Elena was self-contained. It took me a while to realize that might be a problem for me. And the last thing I wanted was to disturb her sense of security.

Elena: And I felt grabby about the experience. I wanted it for myself.

Dick: Maybe I envy you more than I ever acknowledge. What an experience! I tend to run issues out in the abstract. I take pleasure in someone else's accomplishments rather than envy them.

It strikes me that the group was such a special setting for me because it was one of the few places where we knew that someone would listen to the next thing we would say, no matter what it was. We knew it wouldn't be just tolerated, but the attempt to understand would be made in an open-minded way. My confidence in that allowed me to go on to say the next thing...I might not have been able to do that otherwise.

Elena: In other groups, others are always waiting to say their thing.

Dick: It's true. I know in most group situations, I like to be the center of attention. I suppose everyone does. It was much easier to deal with her because I knew that the quality of attention given to each person would eventually be focused on me, too.

I was never bored. People were sharing quite honestly, sharing deep parts of themselves. I found their concerns related to me. I was always learning something from what was happening and so I didn't feel impatient about listening to others.

I had an awful lot of ambivalence about our co-leader, Tom. In particular, about being manipulated—of being plugged into a system that was not of my own making. I'm used to working with systems, but I had a terror getting in touch with my own feelings. Now, I'm more comfortable if someone says, "This process will get you in touch with your emotions."

Leni: Why were you more suspicious of Tom than of me?

Dick: Because Tom was a man. I had to take him seriously. I was used to being manipulated by my mother. I knew how to handle that—or at least I had a system for that. And my father had bullied me.

Leni: Did being in the group help you with the second pregnancy?

Dick: I didn't have a romantic sense about birth this time around. It was a more peaceful, steadier feeling. The earlier group experience was very helpful in helping that happen. It relaxed me. Would I have put earphones on Elena's abdomen unless we had done those exercises dialoguing with the baby? At the time I felt very foolish, writing that letter to the person in the womb. But it was an icebreaker—a party game..Even as I did it, there was a spine-tingling sense that there was a person inside and that I could contact it.

Elena: The exercises did threaten me. I was in therapy. I felt safe there and I didn't want you to threaten that relationship. I was pretty angry with you, Leni, a lot of the time. I felt you shouldn't have been involved in this kind of group leadership because you weren't a professional or credentialed. Tom was, *he* was a doctor. I felt pressured to have this ideal birth. You said I had control. I didn't see that I did. But I valued the male/female co-leadership a lot…it was really important. I had always gone to women to share my feelings. And my therapist was a woman. I liked the fact that Tom was a doctor, even though he wasn't an ob-gyn. It made me feel comfortable and confident. He also shared a lot of himself. And being in the group with fathers and role playing a visit to the doctor with their participation helped me deal with the second birth and the doctor I had this time. Incidentally, he could have done me in but I didn't let him. This time, I had a vaginal birth, even though the first one was a caesarean.

Dick: Tom was a wonderful model for me because he was soft inside. I hadn't given it much conscious thought before the group experiences. My ambition was to feel and to express the feminine part of me. I realized that philosophically I believed that, but in practice I suppressed it. Male role models in my life haven't emphasized that.

Elena: I do think most people have their babies for specific intellectual reasons which may mask the unconscious ones. I never thought about it, but I am a "Show me" person. It's hard for me to take risks. Having a baby and writing a book were great risks. I was struggling with my identity at the time. I didn't feel I had any professional identity; everything was unresolved for me at the time of the group. I kept thinking, how can Leni say she is a professional when *I* can't? She's just working on her doctorate.

Do you remember my dream about the garbage? I was letting go of the need for credentials...finding out who I was.

Dick: It's interesting, Elena, that the book you went on to write paid honor to exactly that "anticredentialed" mode. And that even your therapist was not credentialed.

Elena: It's true—I've changed more in the past five years than in my whole life—no, in the past three years...

Dick: I learn by taking the risk of asking, and through the experience of what happens next.

I think a lot of what's been happening to me began with the group and through the exercises, but it was with the arrival of the child that I began to articulate what was going on, and bring together my intellect and my feelings.

I've never been happier than I am now. It's a challenge and it gives me a lot of energy. That's what therapy is about...freeing energy.

I've gone into therapy since then. I was getting increasingly unhappy in my work. I wasn't allowed to do things I needed to do. I am well on the way now to becoming my own person. I began to suppress my intuitive abilities. Now I know I have to meld and balance these two aspects of myself.

Change is our human goal, our collective striving. What does our role contribute to generate change, to expand, to take on the universe? Customarily, we have thought in terms of physical expansion but it is psychic and psychological as well.

Leni: Dick is changing. He is becoming father to himself as well as to his children instead of simply son to his father.What could be done to make the groups even more effective?

Elena: The tribe doesn't prepare you for parenting. It used to be a secret about motherhood. At least now you can talk about it. A pregnancy group needs to incorporate the post-birth period, too. It's an out of joint time. I tried to escape from it. It would have been nice to anticipate the stresses there as well.

I would like to have a group that followed through the birth and early parenting. In the group we had established a support system and we needed each other afterwards. We needed the people we had shared our deep feelings with, people we could continue to be honest with. We had a hard time at the beginning. Once you have one baby, you forget the early stuff that seemed so important. But the issues remain to be resolved differently with each child.

JEAN AND PAUL

Jean and Paul were in one of the groups. They were divorced two years ago, after twelve years of marriage. Jean has continued her career as an interior designer and has become quite successful. Paul is a management consultant. They continue to live within blocks of each other in New York City so that their son, Josh, can see his father on weekends, and frequently during the week. I visited Jean during the summer after seeing Ria and Eric.

Jean: I didn't know where I was career-wise then, but it's really flourishing now. I'm doing things I really want to do. When Josh was eighteen months old, I got very involved in designing residences and offices and since then I have been very busy.

Paul and I split up when Josh was just over three. Being a single parent is hard and it's been important for Paul and me to maintain a good relationship. We've known each other a long time. We were very young when we met and married.

The value of the group is hard to verbalize; it's much more in the gut than anywhere. There are so many things that only make sense later.

Being in a group with other people who were sharing the same experience put me in touch with the fact that I was part of a universal process. My words then, come back to me now. I had never considered before that my mother had given birth and her mother before her had given birth to her, that it was an endless stream. I suppose it felt like stepping over a barrier to be reunited with humanity—a totality was realized. That's where the group came into it.

Being with others who were going through the same thing, talking about our history...our parents' experience, even our grandparents' experience and about pregnancy and birth as an initiation rite provoked the image of stepping over a barrier. The barrier? Let's see, if it was in a dream, there would be a conveyor belt and several people along the side standing still, then one hopping in every so often...The belt would be endless.

Leni: Is that the life stream?

Jean: Yes. During the pregnancy, I guess I indulged myself so much that I really, really dreamed. I loved my body so much. I loved my pregnancy so much. I think I would want another child, just to be pregnant again. I can't remember feeling bad. I remember feeling how my body felt inside. I think I was more in touch with my center, my physical center, than ever before. And that barrier I talked about had a lot to do with reality, too.

I think I would probably say that the people who were standing there, getting in touch with the flow were women—it was just women on the conveyor belt who were being initiated into the rites of womanhood.

Leni: Could the group be more in touch with that process? Should the groups be just women?

Jean: No, I kept hoping the other men would show Paul how I wanted him to feel. In retrospect (because I wouldn't allow myself to recognize it at the time), I think I became more aware of the differences between my husband and me. I remember feeling upset with some of his views and at the same time feeling guilty at being critical because it should have been a time of togetherness.

Leni: You never got mad.

Jean: Perhaps I might have worked through more of those feelings in the group but I really don't think there was anything to be done about the marriage.

The group experience was helpful. You get some clarity and validation for how you're feeling when you see how others are behaving and responding to you. It was also easier for Paul to see things as they were when he observed it objectively. I guess it was George who really identified with being jealous about what went on in a woman's body. I loved the fact that a man could express those feelings because I'm sure that a lot of men feel that same thing. I liked that Paul could be exposed to how other men felt. It's a major pitfall in a marriage though, because you want your partner to be the way you want them to be instead of seeing them the way they are.

I don't know about the exercises for me. I hadn't had any previous group experience so it felt like a foreign language—a little gimmicky. I would have preferred more talking. I got as much out of the conversation as I did the exercises—that is, looking at my expectations in relation to what others had experienced. It is true that a lot of feelings got stirred up, but there didn't seem to be an outlet for the feelings. Maybe it was just me not being able to deal with my feelings.

Leni: We probably needed to have private sessions with each couple at intervals also, but that would have involved a longer time commitment than you had made.

Jean: Maybe it would be better for everyone to be in private therapy concomitantly, or maybe it would just have been better for me. Now that I am in therapy and have been for three years, I can get in touch with the feelings I had then...I can know how angry I was then at certain times and how painful it was.

Paul and I had very strong feelings for each other, but our marriage didn't work.

I know I would have been absolutely crushed if Paul hadn't been there at the birth. I think if it hadn't been for the group, we would have had a harder time.

What impressed me the most was the way in which each couple predicted the way their birth would be. What that says to me is that each of us has the power to control the experience to some degree. That's the one thing that stands out for me.

It would be nice to recapture the excitement of a second birth by being in another group. People seem so much less intense about a second birth. The group makes it so much more than just having a child, you are brought into the mainstream of society. I know I would be much more carefree about a second child. Right after Josh was born, I remember washing my hands every time I picked him up!

AMY AND DON

Amy has pursued her career as a weaver and works full-time at her studio in downtown Manhattan. Don teaches economics. They take equal responsibility for childcare of their son. They have maintained a friendship with one of the couples from their group.

Don: Even though it wasn't planned, we were delighted. I was very glad it was going to happen. There wasn't any hesitation, no turning back.

Amy: You were less hesitant...you were forty...

Don: Pregnancy is such an "up" time, unless of course, one or the other is against it, though obviously, there are some apprehensions, too. If there are personality issues that get in the way like expectations, desires, it's O.K. for them to get put aside, because giving birth—carrying on the next generation—may be the most important task we ever do and the most important experience of our lives.

The idea that you need support for the pregnancy stage feels like carrying coals to Newcastle.

Leni: It's nice to see that you're now so secure about your fathering abilities, Don, because you sure felt a lot more vulnerable back then. How well do you remember the group? For instance, what about the exercises? Were they useful?

Don: If I think back, I don't remember the exercises. I remember the people very vividly, what they said and how they related to each other. I only remember what we were *talking* about. In particular, what others were talking about, not even what I was talking about...I don't know whether that is selective memory.

Amy: I do recall the exercises—I think they helped us express some problems that were difficult. I remember we had a fight about competing over this child that hadn't even been born yet. There is still some of that between us. However, I think we focus on him rather than competing with each other.

Don: I think that happened long after the birth.

Amy: No, it was there in anticipation.

Leni: Do you remember that when you talked in the group, Don would listen thoughtfully and give you a lot of support? He would sit next to you, quite obviously admiring you, playing with your hair, twirling a stray lock, giving you the very attention that you felt that you weren't receiving?

Amy: I know, that has continued. I realize he spends a lot of time looking at me and I'm not aware of it.

I've been weaving since the birth and I've had my own studio for two years. Leaving school and starting to work by myself was a trauma for me. It was almost impossible to do anything at first. It was physically difficult for me to get my whole self into it and I still don't have my whole self into it, but I'm more into it than I was two years ago. There's just this tremendous fear. It feels like this is the big test...

Leni: You are saying the same thing about fear and the big test, as you did during the pregnancy in relation to the birth.

Amy: Am I? So much of it has to do with lack of information, that's why it was so huge. Every step of the way is in the dark...birth, nursing, childcare.

Leni: Often so much of that information is inside you. It's allowing yourself to know what you already have sensed intuitively.

Amy: I'm starting to have a glimmer of that now, in my work.

Don: The most valuable part of the group was making the whole thing less mysterious, since we had no idea what to expect—particularly in relation to the medical community. Our experience was despicable. The whole idea of deferring to the doctor was the big shock of the whole experience. Because we went through the experience with the group, we knew that our experience was despicable. In the group, you came to trust your own judgment more about what pregnancy should be.

Our problem was with the medical profession...Even today, I still have that problem—I went to a doctor to have him look at a mole...he said it was a wart. When I asked him what the difference was, he said, "I don't have time to explain." The same old stuff, just like Amy's doctor saying she can push till Doomsday and it won't make any difference and not bothering to explain. How dare he say that? Nothing's changed.

As we talked in the group, you had less input, Leni, than any of the people there. I was interested in the psychology of Alan and Dick and Eric and others, but you and Lucy Ann [a nurse] had a lot of information from us, eliciting our feelings but you were the expert and should have been telling us.

Amy: My general memory is one of resentment that we were giving you a lot. I guess it was my fear of being controlled or of losing control over this experience, because it was such a nice pregnancy and because I was so ignorant of the process...and of what happens. Even the childbirth classes seemed to explain nothing, give no variables, no experiences of anyone else. It was really like jumping off a cliff. I knew nothing. But you knew a lot and so did Lucy Ann. You knew doctors, you knew other situations, but you never told me any of that. And you could have. You could have told me, he shouldn't be treating you like this, instead of saying, "How do you feel about him treating you this way? There are doctors who don't treat you like this." But that wasn't your purpose, you were there to transcribe, to take notes.

Leni: Do you remember seeing the videotape in which you two were reporting about your office visits and complaining about your doctor?

Amy: I do remember talking about the doctor all the time.

Leni: We spent a lot of time on the issue of your feelings about your doctor. You didn't seem to want to hear me or others say anything about changing doctors. "Why are you going to that doctor?"...Eric said impatiently one night, "There are better doctors, you are getting fucked over by that doctor." It was said several times at different intervals by many members of the group. And now, years later, as we talk I'm hearing a repetition of attitude and, in fact, the same kind of language you used before.

Amy: What attitude?

Leni: The doctor is the expert; that he knows best. Don said then, "I respect doctors; they know what they are doing." I'm a professional and I respect professional training. All of us "professionals," including Lucy Ann, who was a nurse, and Ria, who was in nursing school, would say, "Look, doctors don't know everything. You may have to shop around until you find one that really suits you." But you seemed to want to stay with the one you had and be mad, instead of switching to someone more satisfying. I recall that very specifically because I was feeling frustrated. I didn't know how far to go with advice, how much to comfort you. I was consciously *not* replacing the doctor as an authority—you were angry at me for not playing into that dynamic, for not taking control. I didn't want to make decisions for you. That was not my role. I was trying to help you hear yourself and trust your own feelings.

Don: The doctor was a forceps man, and we didn't even know what a forceps was.

Amy: I couldn't even conceive of changing doctors. It's one thing to feel that the doctor is fucking you over, another for you to tell me that I should go see this new doctor or recommend someone.

However, it was wonderful to have that companionship in the group; that was great. There were ties formed there. I would have liked us to be even closer to each other, to have been more of a community. I'm glad that I did it. I would have liked to have done more things like the dialogue with the baby. I remember that so vividly. Pregnant women are always communicating with their child, but this was deeper. I really transcended my own neurotic worries, and drew out some realness in me that doesn't come out very often. I think becoming a mother has changed me for the better.

I also wish there had been more touching of other pregnant women. It would have been good for men to have had more touching, too.

ANNE AND SAM

Anne and Sam moved to California after the birth of their first child, Mark. Anne was a management consultant. She's now doing graduate work in medical anthropology, with emphasis on children. Sam is an airlines executive, as he was during the group. They moved because Sam's firm sent him to the west. Their second son, Ted, was born nine months ago. Both children were born at home, one in New York and one in California.

Both Anne and Sam felt that the positive aspect of the group was its effect on the development of their own relationship.

> **Anne:** As I sat and listened to us in the group, I realized that Sam and I had separate lives for the past seven years. Our work took us into different worlds and as we pursued our careers and traveled about we were involved with different people in quite different fields. I hadn't understood how separate we were.

> **Sam:** This was the first important thing we faced together.

> **Anne:** We had to come to grips with working things out in common, doing some problem-solving together. The process of drawing together was very powerful for me and is still quite clear to me six years later. I recall we sat there drawing on one piece of paper. I felt in touch with nature and organic function; I drew a large tree. There was no person in my image, however. When Sam came along and put in the person, I scratched out the figure Sam was drawing. I was annoyed. I didn't want a person messing up my image of nature. Imagine! I realized when I remember those feelings that having people in the group who were further along than I was, helped make my pregnancy seem more real earlier on. I needed to accept it, not continue to feel that it was a movie, and not happening to me.

> **Sam:** I remember that Anne was quite ambivalent in the early months, not about having the baby, which she wanted—but about accepting all the complexities of the social

changes that subsequently occur. It took time to work that through to a comfortable place. The group helped us focus on important things that had to develop in our relationship as a couple so that we would be in a good place to welcome the new person. We began to realize what it is like to have a baby.

We listened a lot to how others felt. There was a rare depth of sharing with the others. We understood more about how we ourselves had been treated and how that patterned our lives. We felt much better prepared as a result. Our relationship is closer than it has ever been.

Anne: In the second birth, I felt Sam's total support. The experience in the group probably helped him do that. And now with our second baby, we sit down and talk about our differences in attitudes about childbearing...We have come together around the children.

Sam: I can't truly recall specific exercises, or even the exercises in general or the feelings I had during them. I did like the structure of the evenings and enjoyed the group. It was very important to us.

Anne: I liked the exercises. In fact, recently I wanted some help to look once again at issues that arose. Some were the same and I wanted to go into them more deeply. I went to various groups for help, tried to start a parent group with fathers as well as mothers. No luck! Finally, I organized a support group which met every third week. When I was trying to plan some sessions for this group of parents, I used some of the exercises from our group and from other exercises I'd had. It's an art to apply them to the right moment. I feel you did that well in our group. I felt they were facilitative.

There is no place to get in touch with the feelings during pregnancy. In childbirth classes, they say education will take care of the fear but they don't deal with it. Letting myself feel vulnerable was my personal task. It was the first time I could let myself do it. I prided myself on my great strength before, out there in the male world. I feel that to be a key issue in the contemporary world—allowing the feelings of vulnerability to be there instead of in control and invulnerable. Surrendering. That's what one learns in therapy or I did, anyway...allowing oneself to be sad, to be in pain, to feel fear...it's all part of life. I recall one in which we focused on a light that circulated around the baby and after we relaxed we were asked to talk to the baby.

It was important to me to deal with the baby as a person, important to deal with its consciousness from the start. It was simple but profound. I have recommended that exercise to many pregnant friends. It's odd to recall all this now. I was surprised at how much more acceptance Sam had for having a child. He connects with the kids on a deep level; he's a good father. He doesn't have a lot of close adult friends, so it's a side I hadn't seen.

I do remember that I didn't feel as close to the group as I wanted to. I think I would have liked more socializing in between. And yet the support they gave us was essential.

We never would have done a home birth without the group. I discovered that I had choices, that it was important for me to arrange things the way I wanted them to be. The group gave us the impetus to design our birth environment as we dealt with all the issues of designing one's birth in the group. Hearing the horrors of others' experiences convinced me that we had to have it at home.

Sam: Now that I look back at our first home birth, I realize that we were so lucky. Things fell into our laps...the compliance of our traditional OB, the support of our two best friends, who were both doctors and offered us their home for the birth which was close to the hospital. In California, the region of home births, strangely, it was hard to find help for the second birth. If we had had to push as hard to organize the first as we did the second, we wouldn't have done it. It was so great the first time that we did persevere.

Anne: I find the women's movement is still putting down motherhood right and left. The most difficult aspect of my life has been integrating my commitment outside the world and inside the domestic realm. The group could help me find my true feelings, which were that I needed to go with family as long as that was necessary, although I didn't get specific help on that issue. But in actuality, I had to hear from a man I really trusted that it was all right to have a family as first priority. My male colleagues were saying to me, "My wife is so miserable. Don't choose to stay home." I'm happy I chose to have a family, and Sam and I are struggling with how we each participate in the domestic realm. The world needs to help men get the joy that is inherent in creating and shaping lives. We're working at the parenting process. We had no idea of what parenting would be like. I now have a whole notion that you develop as the child develops. Things are different in contemporary America.

The transpersonal aspects of birth were closer to me this time, permitting me to feel the spiritual presence. It has been most powerful for me and Sam. We chose a quotation from Lao-Tzu to say it for us for the welcoming of our second child. We wanted something besides baptism which is a ceremony that washes away the sin from the baby. I was feeling just the opposite...how do we keep the purity of this being?

> The breath of life moves through a deathless valley
> Of mysterious motherhood
> Which conceives and bears the universal seed,
> The seeming of a world never to end,
> Breath for men to draw from as they will:
> And the more they take of it, the more remains.
>
> *The Way of Life*, Lao-Tzu
> (translated by Witter Bynner)

We needed you the second time, Leni. I wish we had been able to be with you in a group for that time. You know I called you to see if you could put it together even for a weekend. Let me send you a journal entry from my second pregnancy—the learning goes on, you know.

August 7, starting last trimester: "I want to write about what went on for me about a month ago, after I got back from New York. When I visited good friends there, I was feeling very positive about my life now—the prospect of graduate work, which I've already embarked on and am feeling productive about; the coming baby, which delights Sam, too; Sam and I are at a good level of caring and acceptance; Mark is lovely; our new home is wonderfully restorative, a joy to be in; we are basically healthy; Sam's job is going very well. So I exuded this aura of competence, and genuinely felt it.

"Then I came home, was glad to be home, but realized I was walking around with all this anger—at everyone, even the shopkeepers, other drivers, the whole world, in fact. Just all-pervasive anger.

"I let my irrational self express it, and here's what it said, loud and clear: 'I want to be taken care of.' It was an overwhelming feeling, all pervasive, totally vulnerable and needy. I want a mother and father. I want someone to take care of me at the birth, and before and after.

"Well, I still get in touch with this level of feeling from time to time. Probably I'll never lose it and maybe it's a human dimension. Who says I have to be competent all of the time? I still want to be held sometimes. Mainly, I have to let myself feel vulnerable; just acknowledging the feeling really helps a lot, and it helps connections with other people who are also in need.

"I'm less demanding. I'm closer to Mark and Sam. But it is painful, too.

"I suspect pregnancy intensifies these feelings of vulnerability, though they are always present in us, just usually buried really deep, under the anger and control."

RACHEL AND ALAN

Rachel conceived during the last month of the group and gave birth at a birth center, one of the few in the Pacific Northwest, the region of her own birth. Rachel and Alan have stayed in the Northwest, where Alan has been the doctor for a small community for the past four years. During the period of the group workshop, he was completing his residency in a large New York hospital.

Rachel is busy as a homemaker and helping to develop the farmland they have bought and taking care of their daughter, Susie. When I saw them they were expecting their second child, who was due in six months.

It was eight months after the group had ended when their first baby was born. They called me to share their excitement. They had driven to their birth center at ten a.m. with the majestic sight of the mountains before them. As the sun was setting at five-fifty-five P.M., Susie was born. The birth center was a perfect place for Rachel to give birth.

Rachel: The environment was like a home and full of momentos. Contractions went fast, the midwife was a sweet, beautiful woman, a perfect person to have there. I felt so happy to see her. Alan was there and felt a little jealous and left out because this woman was so special to me. Later we talked about it and it was O.K. The second stage took longer and was a little complicated but it worked out. I felt irritated at some points that the baby was so difficult and disappointed to have to have an episiotomy.

During labor I felt so earthbound, nothing else mattered. It was an all-encompassing experience. Nothing else mattered. Alan didn't matter, just giving birth. I thought at one point, "I'm not getting spiritual enough," but in retrospect, there was a glow about it. I didn't need bells or music. It was extraordinary.

Alan: Early on during labor, I felt she needed a servant, not me, just someone to fetch and carry. I felt resentful. I wanted it to be a peak experience for her. I heard it was such a high, but how do you absorb this life experience in such a little time? But it was magical.

It's difficult to bring ourselves mentally back to that time, to be able to easily discuss the birth group. That emotional state is worlds away. Our lives have changed so much, I am no longer who I was then—my marriage and practice aren't the same and yet it's timely that you have asked us just now, because Rachel's pregnant with our second child—you're one of the few people who know now. We feel that we would like to keep this one a secret for a few months—

something to be experienced just by us at first before we spring it on the grandparents and friends.

Rachel: The first time I was pregnant we were going to be homeless for quite a while and it was quite different. Now we're part of a community and we're going to be around for the next many months.

Alan: Pregnant women get a little of what I get as a doctor. I can't even go to social occasions on the island without being assailed by questions and personal problems—I've started to avoid parties, even though I used to be very gregarious.

Rachel: We had to become secure enough in our relationship to feel O.K. enough about bringing someone else into our family. A lot of my concern was due to the fact that my parents were divorced and that caused me a lot of distrust in relationships. I was finally able to feel confident enough in our relationship to go ahead.

Alan: We both take the idea of marriage very seriously— which made us very frightened of the responsibility that we were taking—in terms of the commitment that we made. Also frightened that if we didn't do it right, it wouldn't work, because all around us people were having trouble with their relationships. At times it seemed like everybody was. There we were even before we had a baby wondering whether it was the right thing to do and it seemed like Rachel didn't get pregnant until it was right for it to happen. Even now, sometimes we wonder...

Rachel: You have to have a firm base because there are all kinds of tests. There's that complication of another person. It does make marriage a lot more difficult. We have moved a lot in time and space, though, by coming to this community. I can't imagine a farther place to be from where we were in Manhattan—in both environment and culture, at least in the United States. It's so different being in a city of several million to being in a town of several thousand... We're still surrounded by water, though.

Alan: We've changed so many of our ideas. Some of our old ideas seem to us so naïve now. That's the way it goes. I was such a radical—a revolutionary—but in becoming a father I realized I didn't want to bring a child up in chaos. It is reminiscent to see young people who are just getting married who are so idealistic.

Rachel: I think I already feel a qualitative difference with this pregnancy. I don't mean that the magic is not there, I'm sure I'll feel the same as I did, but we were on a cloud the first time. We had bought a dulcimer just to play music for the baby while we drove across the country. That's great, but I'm much more practical now.

You asked about how the exercises helped and what impact they had. I remember one in particular. We were acting out going to the doctor's office and stating what we wanted. That helped me a lot because when we came out here I hadn't had any continuous medical care. I had just stopped on the way and had various people examine me. I was about five months pregnant and very healthy. I had a lot of expectations for the birth. Fortunately, I found a birth center out here. I went into the birth center armed with all these questions—and very determined. Working together with the group in New York helped me formulate and verbalize my ideas. Having practice helped. It turned out not to be necessary because the midwife in the clinic was anxious to do what parents wanted.

Alan: When it came to deciding where we would have the baby, I was less anxious to have it in a birth center than in a hospital—the hospitals in this area are not like big city hospitals with their cold, steely environments. Of course, hospitals here are not the same quiet, personal places that perhaps a birth center or home is but they are much more geared towards families and natural childbirth. They have rooms that are set aside for this kind of birth—different from those we had left, where midwives had to be hired furtively in order for women to have babies that way. I'm sure things have changed in other parts of the country by now. This birth center has helped to pioneer new ways. We were fortunate, but even so, I wasn't that eager because I was concerned about the risks.

Rachel: I want to have the baby at the same birth center. But I'm also not that opposed to the hospital. I'd be willing to go look, whereas before I would only have been willing to go if I couldn't have the birth center—I don't feel so threatened by the hospital now, maybe because I know some of the doctors now and I trust them.

Leni: Do you feel different about this pregnancy?

Alan: It's again a transition time—but we'll be living here for some time. We're remodeling our house now and will probably just be taking off the roof and beginning phase two when the baby is born.

Rachel: There's no perfect time to have a baby.

Alan: Getting back to the value of birth groups, I feel that they are specially good for first-time parents. It's like medical students. They are much more fun to have around than residents or doctors because they will have a certain eagerness and interest and curiosity. Also, they have some special issues to cover, and the same thing is true for new parents who are getting together and sharing their ignorance. Those exchanges provide comradeship and a realization that others are going through the same thing. Also, it's helpful to have someone who is experienced like you—in working out and understanding those relationships from a different standpoint—guiding the group.

Rachel: I think a birth group is still important for parents who have more than one child. I have a certain amount of anxiety about this new pregnancy. I wonder how I'm going to do it all. It would be good to talk to other mothers about what they do—it would ease my anxiety.

Alan: Now that you mention it, I can certainly see it would be valuable for us to be involved in another group like that. Maybe even a mixed one with first-timers as well as old-

timers. I feel a qualitative difference between the first pregnancy and this because we focused on that one. I recall it
as a magical, idyllic period.

We started going to your birth group in New York when
we weren't even pregnant—until the end of the group.
Rachel got pregnant just a couple of months before we left
for here. The most important part of that time was that it
was a great transition in our lives. We were negotiating our
relationship to allow ourselves to become a family.

My feelings about life are that love and romance are the
glue that allow almost impossible things to happen between
people. Because otherwise it doesn't make much sense for
people to be together, because everyone's so different they
will never get along completely. Only love and intangibles
like that keep people and families together. The romance
keeps things together while the practical things get worked
out. Now I'm less romantic about having a baby. I can feel
a rekindling of memory of the first time...

Rachel: It's fun talking about it—I now have such a different point of view. I was in awe of it all. I'm not looking forward to having my figure go again. The first time it was
awesome to watch it happen. This time I know what's
going to happen. I'm going to get a big belly. But I know
I'll probably get caught up in the magic again.

Alan: I would like to see a birth group here like we had in
New York. It would force people to turn their TV sets off
and give them a chance to discuss their relationship in front
of other people and get some things resolved that they may
have been putting off. I know we had several of those
issues, though none of them stands out in my mind clearly
at this point. Those meetings produced a lot of emotional
feelings.

We've changed a lot—a group would have a very different meaning right now—I'm sure the issues we would be
bringing up would be much different.

Rachel: At the time, though, having a baby in an unconventional way was going against the trend. I really felt I needed
support—going to the group, reading the books, talking to

the other women to build up that determination that I was going to do it.

Alan: There was a whole gamut of different responses in the group—even though we had similar values and attitudes. Several families from the group had their babies in the hospital, one at home, one at a birth center, for instance. We were all happy for each other and it was the right thing to do it the way we each did it. There was support for the way each couple went to the finish line.

Rachel: You never told people how they should do it. We were just told about the possibilities.

Alan: The group didn't create unrealistic pressures, or claim that everyone should have a home birth. Even though you want natural childbirth, it's possible that you may have to have a C-section. The important thing is to have a healthy baby!

Some larger patterns of response began to emerge from the interviews I collected. Several aspects were striking to me. Six years after the birth of their children, some of the men showed a tendency to minimize the needs and vulnerabilities they clearly felt during the first pregnancy. Their partners, in contrast, vividly remembered how crucial the support groups had been for them. What might be the source of the father's reluctance to acknowledge their need—a reluctance that may make it difficult for men to join a birth group in the first place? Men feel a cultural pressure to be masterful, strong and dependable in the face of their impending parenthood—an honorable impulse, but an impossible demand. This pressure makes it even more difficult for them to express the complex of feelings—ambivalence, envy, rejection—that accompanies pregnancy. In the group, men could share these taboo feelings, but later on, it seemed more difficult for them to admit how frightening and immediate these feelings had been. Other men experienced this vulnerability in ways that allowed them to make a transition to new, deeper and stronger levels of feeling. In contrast, *not one* of the women denied the need for such support groups. Men were agreeable if their wives wanted them to attend, but few felt strong personal motivation to join on their own initiative. It's my hope that a father's psychological participation during pregnancy and birth will come to be seen increasingly as a source of personal gratification for men, and will not be something that is done simply to please their partners.

Another thread that became apparent was the issue of ambivalence toward authority—in this context, the medical professionals. In some cases, parents were torn between the natural desire to be taken care of, giving up autonomy, and the more socially acceptable pressure to decide for themselves and guide their own birth experience. If the ambivalence is not cleared up during the pregnancy, the result can be disappointing—if not disastrously confusing during labor and delivery, with mother and doctor at odds. A birth group can help couples decide what kind of birth they *really* want, and for what reason, and then help them plan for it. For example, there should not be pressure to have a midwife if that is not what the couple truly desires—or to have a home birth. If the choice is not made with full awareness of the pros and cons, they may not be able to handle the responsibility. The important goal is to clarify the personal attitudes and desires of each couple.

Although each couple had their own individual words of praise or criticism for the place of the group in their lives, the overwhelming general impression was that it provided focus during a difficult time.

In sharing feelings and experience, the group became aware of the cultural attitudes with which they were raised— the taboos, the expectations, the limitations, the myths. Exposing these assumptions allowed them to sense the ways in which they were either continuing the same response patterns, rebelling against them, or evolving a personal value system.

Most people remembered the birth itself much more than the pregnancy's less focused feelings, although as we met once a week for months, there were more emotions to express than we had time for. Once the pregnant period was over, it seemed that those passionate concerns of pregnancy were quickly replaced by new sets of equally compelling parenting concerns.

In subsequent groups, I acted more assertively and sought backup support from another therapist when needed. Working with a male partner was also extremely important for two reasons. It allowed one of us to sit back and observe while the other was involved, and it allowed couples to view us as supportive or nonsupportive parent figures—as both the good and bad mother and father. I feel that directness and honesty for the leaders and from the group leads to expansion and growth as long as it is within a caring and supportive context. Problems that seem critical and need more private time can be handled by a consulting therapist. In fact, I would recommend each couple have a private session with the leaders once every few weeks as well.

Research on the emotional aspect of birth has demonstrated that those who allow themselves to confront their deepest conflicts before the birth have an easier time afterwards. We will know more as we explore further. We are only beginning to collect data on this particular family transition, and even as we do, the structure of contemporary family life is changing.

In my discussion at the onset of the group meetings, I had emphasized that we would deal with emotional issues relevant to pregnancy. It was to be an exploratory group—not a therapy group in the generally accepted sense of that word. In planning such groups, I realize that it is important to be very specific about the goals and psychological boundaries you wish to set for yourselves.

Each couple in such groups is working at a creative task, trying to shape their experience, experimenting with new attitudes and behavior, making choices that might allow a more harmonious flow with the natural order of the universe—"man in nature" as opposed to "man over nature." It can be an enriching process, as Sam said:

> We witnessed dramatic changes in the lives of each couple,
> not only around the subject of birth.

However, experiencing feelings in the group was by no means a panacea. Anne added:

> Not everything was solved in the group. My own weakness-
> es persisted and persist still. A couple can't rearrange the
> total pattern of their lives in five months. I spent thirty-two
> years becoming who I am and learning to behave the way I
> do. Learning a new way wasn't about to happen overnight.
> However, the group showed us a way of approaching the
> experience of pregnancy and birth—which *did* thoroughly
> rearrange our lives!

> **Sam** said philosophically: You can *plan for* any kind of
> birth, keeping in mind that what actually happens may not
> be under your control or the perfect control of anyone else.

Changes, transition, process. New roles, new status, new responsibilities to confront. Yet, in touch with the universalities of the transition, everyone connected to the same source, fed by the same wellspring. As the group shared deeply with others, as they listened sensitively, it became apparent that we were connected. Another's story was one's own, another's insight clarified one's own dilemma.

And no matter what a couple's feelings are about their baby's birth, it is crucial to move onward from the birth experience into the next stage of life's continuum, the new relationship with their child outside the womb. Its parents' love and caring attention are *the* most important aspect of a baby's life.

Each passage in the life cycle is part of the continuum; each with its own insights and tasks.

7

GUIDELINES FOR STARTING
YOUR OWN GROUP

Mothering and fathering may be instinctual,
but as each change in our world further
rips the ancient web of human life,
love and instinct need a bit more help.
—Marshall Klaus, Oakland Children's Hospital
(Oakland, Ohio)

There are, of course, innumerable ways to design pregnancy support groups. The characteristics and needs of the group will be the defining factors. If you want to be the initiating force, here are some suggestions for finding others to join you and ways to run the sessions.

You may have friends who are also expecting a child who will be interested in helping to establish a group. Perhaps you may even decide to form a supportive foursome. Two couples I know did just that. Their story follows in this chapter.

Establishing a larger group of eight to ten committed couples is probably more to the point, however. Canvas your pregnant friends and friends of friends. Or your obstetrician, family physician or midwife may furnish a list of prospects. Another source may be your local school, church or the hospital where you get prenatal care. Posting a notice on a community bulletin board or a local health food store, infant clothing exchange, or book-store may work too. It's helpful if members of the group live in reasonably close proximity so that there isn't too much travel time involved. You know best the opportunities in your community.

You might emphasize that it is to be a group for first time parents or second or third pregnancies since it is beneficial when everyone is speaking from a similar experience. However, as you can see from the comments of the parents described in this book, those having their second child also derived great benefit from being with first-time parents.

Childbirth educators are a good source and can help form a group by referring couples from their classes.

If you think you want more experienced guidance, a child-birth counselor might be interested in leading the group or you can enlist a therapist to run it or perhaps only come assist at thorny times.

Begin the group early in the pregnancy, as early as possible, allowing the many months ahead for unfolding and working through problems. Usually preparation classes for labor and delivery start in the seventh or eighth month so it is wise to start this intensive support earlier. Even so, there may not be enough time for all you want to deal with.

Is there an ideal size for a pregnancy support group?

It is preferable not to have the groups too large—eight to ten members. Remember to take into account that not everyone will be able to attend every meeting. Small groups allow more time to be heard and known. "Air time" is important. Trust and inti-macy develop more easily among fewer people and that's an essential element in the group process.

I've contacted five interested couples. We've agreed to meet once a week. What do we do next?

You can just plunge in using this book as a guide. Other helpful literature is listed in the bibliography. Trust yourselves. The success of consciousness-raising and other groups in the past has demonstrated the value of self-led groups; people involved in the same experience have great wisdom and insight to offer to each other. Self-led groups may develop differently from those led by a therapist or childbirth educator. Therapists will probably be able to lead participants deeper into the issues that emerge.

If you decide to work on your own, you might find a standby counselor who will be available for backup support or individual sessions when needed. Issues can arise for an individual or a couple that require more time or skills than the group can provide. This person who may be male or female, should preferably be a parent his/herself and have some experience with this rite of passage and its tumult.

Do we really need to begin with a weekend session as you recommend?

Whenever possible, I suggest that you begin with a weekend intensive workshop. You can move down the road faster as you experience each other in more depth. Bonds can more readily develop. Getting to know each other is a process that needs time. You can get a feel for each other's personalities and be able to sense the pace for each participant's unfolding process. Some of us are able to open up and share more freely than others. Respect each other's timing.

Having a weekend together, enjoying comparative freedom from responsibility before the baby comes can be a bonus. If a weekend away is not possible, two consecutive days make a difference.

After the weekend, the group can agree on a meeting night and commit to a schedule. Commitment is important for each couple needs to be able to depend on ongoing support.

Whether or not you can arrange a weekend workshop, it helps to start the session with a design similar to the format that follows. Let your group develop gradually without pressure or expectations so that everyone feels it is a safe, protective environment in which to share feelings.

What should we do at the beginning?

Arranging for each couple to host a meeting in turn is a good way to learn more each other too. It gives everyone a chance to be relaxed in their own environment. As the body is an envelope for the psyche so is the house the next concentric circle of the psyche. It's conducive to the kind of sharing and intimacy that needs to develop.

If you are sharing the leadership of the group among yourselves, decide before you begin which of you can best lead the session that evening. Emphasize love and compassion. Be sparing with heavy criticism and judgment. Remember this is a *support* group.

Begin the session as early in the evening as possible and hold to a definite ending time. Not only do pregnant women wear out but their partners do as well. The session should not run on and on. Two to three hours is a good length. Clear away coffee tables or any furniture that creates psychological barriers between members of the group. Be aware of the elements in the environment that will support the process. Flowers, for example, unconsciously remind people of nature's creative capacity. Clear the room so that there's space for group exercises. Soft indirect lighting helps; bright enough, however, for everyone to see each other's subtle shifts of facial expression and body language. A tape recorder or record player are important additions.

Honor this time. Create a quiet space for this work. Take the phone off the hook. If possible give yourselves a quiet time at home before the meeting to clear the day's activities.

Begin each session with a relaxation exercise (a meditation or breathing exercise). An initial period of relaxation and focused breathwork loosens everyone up and facilitates discussion. Be sure to give directions for the exercises slowly; a lot happens in between spaces. Use soft music such as "Creative Visualization" by Shakti Gawain to create a calming environment. After five to ten minutes, let people share what they were feeling during the exercise if they want to. Some participants will have had a rich experience. Others may have a more abstract experience and want it to remain personal and private.

Move on to another exercise, a more thematic one. Let the concerns of the evening determine structure, especially if there are urgent issues. When something powerful is happening for one person, a couple, or for the group itself, scuttle the planned exercise and talk, or improvise an exercise that feels right for the situation. The focus will usually be relevant for others as well as for the couple with the problem. Even if you feel you understand their problem and perhaps a solution, don't push people faster·than they want to go. Most of us know our limits. We create our defenses for good protective reasons, they need not be penetrated by others in an insightful moment. Nor should they be. Not until the layer under the defensive skin can acclimate to the light of day.

Explore ways to interact. Be creative. Be honest but remember to be sensitive, kind, compassionate. Follow your feelings. Trust your intuition. Use metaphor, use imagery, use poetic forms, use whatever works for you to release inchoate feelings. Listen with your hearts as well as your minds.

Useful questions after an exercise may be:

- What's happening for you right now. What are you feeling?
- What just happened?

As different themes emerge, different exercises will be appropriate. Also, themes may not arise in the order I have listed. The order is not significant and the dynamics of each group will differ. Basic themes will arise over and over, perhaps in response to different issues than before. Use the same exercise more than once to evoke new insights.

The exercises I have suggested may feel too formal an approach or seem to be manipulative or mechanical. Give them a try. They usually catalyze deeper levels of emotions than can be tapped by simply talking. The emotions once invited will continue to be expressed.

Films can be good. Try your local video store. After about an hour and a half, take a break, stretch, walk around, have some refreshments. After fifteen minutes or so gather back into your circle. Don't lose the momentum and intensity of the group work in casual conversation and socializing, pleasant as that may be. Save that for later.

Move gently into the sharing process. It is easier for some than others. Some people are eager to share their innermost thoughts and feelings, others are reluctant, talking more time to establish trust. Even discussing these differences is grist for the mill and a good place to start examining underlying causes. Be sensitive to issues of confidentiality between partners. Shock treatment isn't supportive. It's a good idea to check out touchy points before they're aired before the whole group. As the group develops, trust will be established. At the beginning, opt for a safe environment.

I've only been able to find one other pregnant couple where both the partners are interested. Can we function effectively as a group?

Definitely. There are no limitations on what you can accomplish. More isn't necessarily better, only different. The important thing is your willingness to air your feelings and concerns.

I'm a single woman, thirty-five, who has decided to have a child on her own. How do I fit in? I desperately need a support group.

You're not alone! Your doctor or people at the local women's clinic will surely know of other women who've made decisions similar to yours, who also need the support and encouragement you are wisely seeking. As more women decide to have children on their own, there will be more demand for prenatal groups composed of partners who may simply be close friends, whether female or male. Ideally, this friend will be the person who will be helping out at the time of your baby's birth, so that you can begin to develop the kind of deep trust and intimacy that you need during the final stages of pregnancy, labor and delivery.

Variations on the basic group
Separate strands: a women's group, a men's group

For each parent, reevaluating one's self-image, understanding one's changing identity and confronting one's insecurities are an intrinsic part of the workshop. If women have little opportunity to express their conflicting emotions during pregnancy, men have far less. One way to encourage men to practice expressing their pregnancy-related feelings in a "safe" environment is to begin an evening by letting the men and women meet in separate groups for the first half of the evening. After the break, couples can get together and share what happened.

In my experience, this variation was an important source of new information for the men and women who participated. They found that they really needed intimacy with and expressions of support from their own sex as well as from their partners. They needed to know which concerns were personal to them alone, which were common to other men or women and which issues were equally relevant to both sexes. There were charged subjects, such as sex and money and power, which elicited different responses depending on the gender makeup of the group. It was crucial for these differences to be acknowledged by discussing them in the larger group, to reach a deeper understanding between couples. The results from my workshops were particularly illuminating and I include some of this material here to show you the potential insights that can be gained from this variation.

It was fascinating to see the unexpected direction taken by the women. Not babies, not personal appearance or sexuality, but work and career were the "forbidden" subjects that the women gravitated towards among themselves.

Three of the women had been working in professional careers and had become quite independent and respected in their fields. They feared that motherhood and domesticity would force them into a restricted and dependent position. An animated discussion took place, often with all the women talking at once and then laughing at themselves. Alone with other women, they talked spontaneously and passionately, interrupting each other constantly, expressing feelings, affection and strong attitudes. With the men, however, they were more controlled and self-effacing, usually allowing their partners to take the dominant role, or even to speak for them, as if responding to an unspoken social norm.

With each other, they expressed passionate concern about their future, about the fear of losing their status as real people, about exchanging their present identities for anonymous ones, as they drowned in a morass of unending, repetitive daily duties. They feared the loss of their hard-won competence in what they referred to as the real world. They were afraid it would suddenly vanish, convinced from what they saw around them that the privileges and satisfactions they enjoyed in their professional lives would be exchanged for a narrow world of domestic drudgery in which there was little feedback or acknowledgment for their competence and creativity. Fears of isolation were .expressed. In fact, they were already beginning to feel devalued, unseen, unloved. Of course, they realized that they were gaining something intrinsically valuable by having a baby; nevertheless they were also poignantly aware of what they might be losing.

Why couldn't they talk openly with their partners about their concerns for their careers, their passion about their work and about getting ahead?

Just as nonpregnant women may find it difficult to be work-centered, independent and yet nonthreatening around men, so pregnant women, who have simply crossed a physiological bridge, find themselves in the same psychological bind. Indeed, their problem is intensified by yet another layer of cultural attitudes. In their pregnant state, they may feel a subtle but powerful social injunction to be obsessed with the welfare of their baby and the glories of impending motherhood, instead of their careers. For them, pregnancy amplifies the conflict between wanting to be "womanly" and "professional" at the same time.

Anne was the most concerned, and often had dared to confront the issue in the mixed group. This evening she was very active in the discussion, among the women.

Anne: I'm on a kind of seesaw a lot of the time. Some of the time I feel really trapped. I'm afraid to share this with Sam. And I extend this to men in general. I feel that the glowing motherhood image is what I ought to be feeling and I'm afraid or reluctant—to tell the truth. When I discovered I was pregnant, I didn't tell Sam for three days.

Leni: What would happen if you told the truth?

Anne: My fantasy is that Sam would say, "You're going backward. I've wanted a child for so long, you've resisted for so long and now we're going back to that place. I thought you'd finally left it." Then he would dredge up all the bad stuff we would get into around having a child. Anyway, it's irrelevant because I *am* pregnant.

That theme ricocheted around the room; nearly everyone identified with it. It also incorporated other themes, like ambivalence, dependency, and fears of being an incompetent mother.

Anne: When I think of what is overwhelming me, I don't think it's the birth itself. It's the results of birth. Will I be able to do it? Will I be good at it? Will I feel that I am carrying most of the responsibility? What will happen to Sam and me? Will I feel trapped?

Elena: I understand. I feel that in giving up "work" I'll become a worthless person. I've swallowed the male value system whole. I realized I felt sorry at one point for a woman in my office who left to have a baby.

Anne was particularly concerned about the upcoming career change in her life, since Sam was being transferred to the California branch of his company and she would be forced to leave her excellent job as a result. Their situation demonstrated the stereotypical contrast between men's and women's commitments to careers or raising families.

Anne and the others wanted to continue to develop as whole persons, they wanted the continued respect they had earned in their fields and the added stimulation of the male-female community they had grown used to in their daily work life. They feared that the breadth and scope of the world in which they moved would be diminished. Ria knew she wanted to experience that world, too, but as yet had no taste of it and—now that she was pregnant—worried that she might never be able to realize her goals.

> **Anne:** It's tough. We're going to become dependent housewives, not earning our own keep. I don't want to be caught in the backwater of domesticity, and yet I want to take care of the child myself.

Another side of the coin was expressed by Rachel.

> **Rachel:** We have an opportunity to drop out for a while and go back later. It's something men who are on the responsibility treadmill lack.

But the anxiety was there; the women felt it, and voiced it. It fed other feelings of uncertainty. I'm giving up so much to be a mother—but will I even be good at it? Am I going to be the perfect mother? Who's requiring me to be? My mother? My husband? Society? Who will I be when I'm a mother?

> **Amy:** Several days ago, I was in a vicious mood. All of a sudden, it dawned on me that I was getting back at Don for making me pregnant. At one point, I asked him why he thought I was acting like this. He came right back and said that it was because he had impregnated me. I was amazed! It came to both of us in a flash.

> **Elena:** I understand that. I was in a similar place. I get mad at Dick for some dumb thing and then resent the baby. I went through a phase when I wouldn't drink my four glasses of milk a day. Dick would pick up on that and keep track of my milk intake. That hit me because I began to feel that he was no longer caring about me but only was concerned about the baby.

It was an animated, intense discussion that exposed strong feelings and only the time constraints and the plan to join the men interrupted it.

THE MEN'S GROUP

Fears about parenting consumed the men, too, we were to discover when we came back together, though different cultural pressures hooked them. Most of them looked forward to the pleasure of a family, but they were apprehensive as well. Although they realized that their world would be enlarged by a child in their lives, they, too, had a fear of being trapped, of becoming domesticated, of losing their "freedom." "It's scary—is it worth it?" "Will I be able to support them? How much do I want to be involved?"

Sharing the concerns with each other gave the men emotional support as it did the women. It allowed them to confront parenting issues outside the boundaries of the marriage relationship and they began to relate to each other in a more trusting way. Although their discussion centered around child care issues and the changes in self-images that would be involved, it took quite a different turn from the women's discussion.

> **Don:** Since my teaching load will be small next year, I am going to have a lot of free time. I will have the major role with the baby while Amy is going to school. I love the idea. I have fantasies of working with the baby nestled against me.
>
> **Eric:** Suppose the baby starts interfering with what you're doing?
>
> **Don:** I assume that it will interfere. But if I start out with the idea that my working hours are being cut by two-thirds anyway, I'm already ahead.

They talked about the difference in male and female roles from their vantage point.

Alan: I have this idea, perhaps old-fashioned, that the baby is a woman's responsibility, her career. I don't think I'd enjoy or be able to spend that much time with the baby...

Eric: Do you see yourself changing diapers? Getting up in the night? Raising the kid?

Alan: I'll approach it as a sacrificial gesture.

Fantasies reverberated around the room until Tom, as leader, focused the talk.

Eric: I'm in the same position as Don and I've sort of had reality thrown in my face. It hasn't made me negative but it just seems very real.

I don't plan to work at all next year and Ria will be working. I'll be writing my dissertation so in a sense I'll be working, but it won't be at a steady job with steady hours like now. So a lot of the responsibility of child care will be mine. I'll have to work out a work schedule with my library time, too. But, like you, Don, I've really been looking forward to this, saying I'm going to be super-father and this is a great thing for men to be getting into. Then I talk with my friend, who feels very much the same way. He's finding it all-consuming. He doesn't get too much sleep at night. He's getting up to share the feedings, too.

My friend feels he's gone through a postnatal depression as a new father...he's overwhelmed. My friend was saying that he think as men assume more responsibility they are going to be experiencing the postpartum blues, too. He sees men taking on all the downbeat feelings about role change that women have been saddled with, being confined, at home all the time with the child, losing their freedom, handling a new set of responsibilities. It hits me very personally right now!

Alan: Can you imagine anything more depressing? And yet, I think I'll get a lot of satisfaction from being with my child, from enjoying it, but not from changing diapers. I'll get it from seeing the child develop and from establishing a rapport with it. I do look forward to directing the child, you know, his likes and his dislikes, but as far as rearing the child...

Eric: What do you suppose rearing really is?

Nick: Well, disciplining the child and changing his diapers—the negative aspects...

Don: You know, as you were talking, I was reminded that my father was such a remote figure during my whole life. It bothered me a lot when I confronted that in psychoanalysis. For a time, I was so angry at my father when I realized what had actually happened. Maybe that's why I am leaning over backward in anticipation, saying to myself that I am going to be the best father that ever was and spend a lot of time with my child. I'm looking forward to it, and you're right, I drop out of my head all of the negative parts of it.

When the two groups merged later that evening, there was a sense of awkwardness, a little like the embarrassment we experienced at our first mixed teenage social.

Alan: Well, what did you women talk about?

Amy (laughing): You go first.

We traded impressions and insights gained from the separate discussions.

Amy: It's interesting that we women had a difficult time coming up with positive feelings and it seems as if the men did that very easily.

In a shocked tone Don said, "Positive feelings about the baby?"

It was funny to look back on that scene and see the reversal of concern that was exhibited. It was as if the women (like men in a classic stereotype) had retired separately to the library with their brandy to talk about "important things" like careers, while their partners repaired to the bedroom to discuss the children, the chores, and the responsibilities of daily existence. It was even funnier when we discovered that indeed the men had done just that—that concern with the subject of rearing children and child care had absorbed their attention.

Why was it easier for the women to "talk jobs" and the men to "talk babies" when they were in groups of their own sex? One explanation may be that expressing one's deeply felt concerns in certain areas in front of one's partner may be interpreted as threatening, competitive behavior. This is especially true when the roles within the relationship are being severely tested. It is difficult to transcend cultural stereotypes even in the *absence* of a baby, and sorting out one's new roles after the child's arrival is an even more difficult task. While trying to understand our attitudes during this period, we may give out confusing double messages: a pregnant woman may be saying nonverbally, "Stay off my turf," while actually saying, "Help me share the burden." Men, too, may feel this same ambivalence when anticipating the role of breadwinner and father.

As fathers in the group became more intimately involved in their own reactions to the pregnancy, they were able to consider their caretaking role during the pregnancy, labor and delivery from a less defensive position. They began to sense their unique and important personal roles in the enterprise of creating and caring for a baby.

Like Eric, they became more involved with fathering questions in their everyday exchanges with others. They found themselves initiating conversations about babies and child care with other men at work. It was new for them to put themselves forward in that way. Participating in the pregnant period and in the birth and child care afterward was the beginning of a lifetime commitment, and reflective of changing cultural attitudes that encourage a more equitable and involved role for fathers.

TWO IS A COUPLE, FOUR IS A GROUP

Groups don't have to be large formal entities. They can be four friends getting together spontaneously to satisfy needs that are emerging for the first time. Many couples, unable to find the support system they wanted in their community, have designed their own. One couple I know started even before conception. Nancy and Bill had been living together for several years before they married. She had been married before and had a child from her first marriage. It was Bill's first marriage. Nancy, a nurse, was back in school getting a master's degree in psychology; Bill, an ex-lawyer, was starting a consulting business in conflict resolution. They lived in Los Angeles.

Although they had been talking about having a child of their own, she had been putting it off. She felt many of the circumstances would have to be different this time. She observed that her friends were feeling as unsupported during their pregnancies as she had felt the first time, and she knew she wanted much more than that. When her closest friend in her master's program confided that she too wanted to get pregnant, she began to reconsider.

> These were to be second children for each of us, and we knew we needed more support during pregnancy than we'd had the first time. We'd each thought about having another child, and it occurred to us that if we had them together, we could establish a mutual support system—over and above that which our husbands could give us. Originally, the idea that our husbands needed support, too, never occurred to us.

Both conceived within a month of each other. They were delighted. They spoke to each other every day.

> We were like two rolypoly children as our pregnancies advanced. We were ironic with each other; we could do that with each other. We could laugh at ourselves together.

The support system grew into a foursome as the wives and husbands met for dinner once a week, and the social occasions gradually turned into marathon parent-consciousness sessions. They would start at seven and each would have his or her turn to talk. Throughout the pregnancy they continued to meet once and sometimes twice a week. They found it helpful to know that the other couple was encountering the same problems and that they weren't abnormal. For the men it was especially good:

> Pete and I started to get close when we discovered how much we had in common. Men have trouble talking about emotions, but we could share our desperation and hear what the other had done in the same situation.

They found the dynamics of their situations to be very similar:

> We'd hear Kate and Pete working through something and say to each other, "That won't happen to us," and then—WHAM—a month later we'd be into the same emotional tangle.

They shared feelings about everything as it occurred, from social concerns to sexual intimacies, comparing experiences and reassuring each other.

These four friends found they all needed a lot of help, since so much was going on all the time and in such intense ways. In the vacuum that existed, they designed something for themselves; they reached out for each other and created a new support system which was very positive for each of them. The best part, according to Bill, was:

> The foursome made it possible for me. I needed to know that what I was going through wasn't unique—I needed to talk to another man about my man problems, and about my woman problems to another woman besides my wife. It allowed for *all* kinds of combinations of interactions. We were not simply locked into our little system.

And to Nancy:

> Everything was allowable, sayable, nothing was forbidden when we got together. Our pregnancy was not isolated outside our lives but was woven in. This human event was part of our ongoing lives and did not separate us.

VERY LARGE GROUPS

There may be times when you would like to lead just one session for a very large group, such as a Lamaze class or the PTA or a church club, or simply for people interested in becoming more aware of what goes on during pregnancy and childbirth. I have developed an exercise which seems to work well with groups as large as fifty to two hundred people, although it is also effective in ones as small as ten. It is a guided fantasy in which participants are led through the pregnancy, labor, and delivery. By choosing to play the role of father, mother, or baby in family units of three, each person senses the feelings that may be experienced during childbearing. (See Exercise No. 20, Guided Fantasy of Pregnancy and Birth, Chapter 8.) By now, hundreds of people have participated in this exercise under my direction, and many have told me immediately afterward or in later letters that the experience was extremely powerful for them.

One lovely letter arrived from an older man, a professor of education in the Southwest, who had been present at the birth of his grandchild after having attended a conference in Chicago where I had led a large group through the guided fantasy. His account, partially reprinted here, is a striking example of the possibilities for growth that new attitudes toward birth offer us— as a society and as individuals.

> Two years ago I attended your workshop on the rites of birth. An experience I had at role-playing the birth of a child gave me an unexpected insight into my own behavior as a father of seven children. The particular behavior in question was a form of flight during the birth of my children. For all seven children I felt a great need to get away from the pain, away from the blood, away from the birth. Sometimes I fell asleep, sometimes I had to be home to attend to the other children. The first time the labor was so interminably long that I just had to get out of the hospital for a walk. During those times (1950-1964) fathers seemed to be accessories anyhow, especially during the actual birth. The physician and medical persons did all the delivery tasks, and then the mother and baby were taken home to begin the new routine. I had become proficient at helping once all were home and I was, in my own mind, a good father. Hence the flight behavior wasn't of concern to me until the advent of a new era, that of natural childbirth and

home births. (I realize, of course, that these had occurred at other times and places but had not been part of my conscious world.) I became aware of the new era through reading and visiting with younger people who were involved in the natural childbirth movement. I had liked the idea; I had intellectually accepted it. However, until I went to your workshop, I had not recognized my earlier fears and attendant flight behavior. So now the question arose in my mind, "Could I now be a father in attendance?"

As I expressed these thoughts to you at the time, I began to feel both guilt and frustration; guilt, in that I had run so many times; frustration, now that both my spouse and I are sterile and I would not be able to test my courage as a father in attendance. You were quick to suggest that a positive way out of both the guilt and the frustration was to help educate my sons so that they would not have the same fears, or at least help them be aware of their fears.

Last summer our son and daughter-in-law announced that they were expecting a baby and that they were planning a home delivery. I was delighted! My wife, the grandmother-to-be, a public health nurse who works full-time with high-risk pregnancies, was considerably less enthusiastic. However, she was outwardly very supportive, helping in any way she could to prepare for the birth.

The mother and father-to-be checked out the idea with a number of persons and they quickly found that some people were extremely fearful of, some even hostile, toward the home birth. Others were very supportive. To maintain their own positive approach to it all, they decided to tell only a few of their plans. Late in the pregnancy they checked with an obstetrician who was willing to deliver the baby at the hospital should it be necessary. That gave added assurance to them and us.

My wife and I began to plan for our vacation to coincide with the expected birth date. As a matter of fact, after talking it over with the parents-to-be, we decided it would be better to be with them after the birth, rather than going for the birth only to find that the baby was late and having to return to work without seeing the baby or the birth. I was still coping with the fear of being there at the birth, even though I could say I wanted to be there—so the idea of going a little later was appealing. My spouse seemed to feel the same way. We kidded, however, with lots of people about going to help in the delivery.

As it turned out, we arrived two days before the baby was born and were able to stay four days afterwards.

Tuesday morning, January 3, at 12:30 A.M., our son Stan woke us, saying "Jo think the baby will be here soon, will you please join us?" The moment we walked into the room we could see the baby's head emerging. I watched Jo's face, Stan's hands and the baby's head, then body. Jo was obviously pushing, but there was no sign of pain on her face—when the baby made the final lunge Jo smiled in relief. The greatest miracle of all, to me, was that almost immediately after emerging from his mother, the baby began to breathe. There was no slapping, no holding by the feet (both of which I had in my mind as part of the ritual); he just began to breath. Then he peed, then defecated, then cried. (I couldn't swear to the order of the last three.) Within seconds the baby was fondling his face on his mother's breast and shortly afterwards sucking. During all of this I did have enough presence of mind to look at my watch. It was 1:25. It had all happened in less than an hour.

The next day I began to reconstruct the experience, bringing to mind my thoughts and feelings during the birth. I had maintained my calm during the entire birth, sufficiently to observe others, to observe the plants, to remember the conversations. I was not nauseated by the blood or the afterbirth. I had wondered earlier if I would be. The notion that I had carried for many years, that pain was a necessity, was dispelled, as was the mystery of boiling water. The fact that family members, including children, were in the room during the delivery changed my vision of doctors and nurses dressed in green and white being the only appropriate witnesses of a birth. The children, four and eight, took the birth as a matter of fact. Jesse, the baby's four-year-old sister, was concerned that she also have some of her mother's attention. She was soon in her mother's arms. The eight-year-old boy said to me the next day, "Why isn't Jo up and eating at the table? She has already had her baby."

Three days later at the supper table we were still marveling at the beauty and normality of the birth. To what human efforts could we attribute the successful delivery? Both Jo and Stan had, almost from the time of conception, planned for the home birth; they had discussed every aspect of it. The fact that it was Jo's second baby gave her additional insights. They had really refused to accept negative what-if kinds of concerns from others. They didn't tell great-grandmother about their intentions because they were concerned about her excessive worry and fear. (I am still not sure how she feels about it, except that she is delighted that the baby is safely here and that Jo is also healthy.) They discussed the birth with the children and the other adult in the house, and finally they sought out a supportive physician who was willing to deliver the baby should there be complications requiring that they go to the hospital. He in turn knew of a pediatrician who was willing to examine the baby three days after birth.

Finally, and probably most importantly, Jo was truly in touch with her body, her feelings and her intuitions. She "knew" it was going to be all right. She never expressed a doubt. She also believes she would have felt, intuited, known, had a normal birth not been in the making. Furthermore, she recognizes that this is not necessarily the way to go for others.

I must say that being such an integral part of the birth, in view of my earlier fears, was one of the highlights of my life to this point. I learned so much; I felt such joy, experienced such beauty. I might put it this way: This experience at once took much of the mystery out of birth and added infinitely to the mystery of life! Or—my grandson's birth was my own rebirth.

The Gift

Each of you is imbuing your unborn child with the qualities of your personality. Some of these qualities pass through you from your forebears. In this meditation, think of a quality in you that you most respect. It may be your ability to care for others, your patience, or your sense of humor, or your ability to sing or draw, or your strength or your willingness to risk.

Lie down in a comfortable position; move closer to your partner if you are doing this meditation together. Father, place your hand over the womb, over your baby. Mother, place your hand over your partner's.

Take a deep breath and let it go. Inhale and exhale: become aware of the rhythm of your breathing, become aware of your partner's breathing, gently breathe in harmony with each other. Inhale, exhale:...breathe gently in harmony with your baby until you are all breathing as one, each a part of the shared life that is unfolding for you as a threesome. Take another deep breath and let it go.... Breathe love through your heart and into the heart of your baby.

Offer your baby a gift today; open your heart and give it your love. Open your thoughts now and offer your baby one of the qualities you treasure most in yourself. Each day, you can offer a different gift, a gift from you, a gift of yourself. Then when your baby is born, it will be surrounded by your most beloved qualities. Think now of the gift you would like to give today and offer it to your baby...

8

THE ENVIRONMENT OF BIRTH

Those who would take over the world and manage it,
I see that they cannot grasp it;
for the world is a spiritual (vessel)
and cannot be forced.
Whoever forces it spoils it.
Whoever grasps it loses it.

—*Lao-tzu*   *29*

Few parents are prepared for the enormous impact a baby will have on their lives. Although they may expect some inconvenience and personal restrictions in their lives, they often discover more complex emotional difficulties than they expected during the course of pregnancy.

How can we make this period of profound physiological and psychological change easier? It is a vital task representing a crucial investment in our national future. It is a rite of passage to be honored and enjoyed as a period of personal growth, not simply as a passage to be endured in isolation and frustration, hoping for the best.

Acknowledgement of the discrete stages of pregnancy as current research defines them enables us to understand this transition and to give support sensitively and effectively to both parents and developing child. As research has demonstrated, the value of sensitive consideration to the baby developing in the womb is of utmost importance. Talking about feelings, fears, and the realities of imminent parenthood with other pregnant couples in support groups provides a sustaining foundation on which to develop as parents of a new family; and as couples do, they have the opportunity to deepen their previous understanding of themselves and their world. In an environment of trust they can develop confidence in their unique intuition and their ability to make good decisions for themselves.

As other cultures have before us, we are recognizing that the process of becoming parents is a profound transitional crisis in family development, a period with its characteristic patterns, a rite of passage that heralds a new state for everyone involved. Honoring this journey and acknowledging the feelings and emotional conflicts that it presents enables everyone to celebrate it as an important turning point instead of fearing or denying it.

Writer Ken Wilber describes crisis as "an unfamiliar level of excitement." My goal in my groups was to make the unfamiliar familiar. I wanted to empower parents to be able to transform this period of crisis into one of opportunity. I believed that, by joining with other pregnant couples in a supportive workshop environmen we could loosen the social and psychological knots.

In reviewing what has happened in the ten years since my dissertation in 1974 and the publication of my first book, *The World of the Unborn*—and forty years after I had been pregnant with the first of my three children—I am aware of another swing of the pendulum. Attitudes and practices have changed once again and undoubtedly will change many more times in the future.

The changes have basically been retrogressive. We trail behind every industrial country in the world in the attention paid to family needs. However, it is my hope that in the coming years a psychological support structure will guide parents-to-be and give foundation to the ever-changing shifts in attitude. As social change continues to sweep our country and the high divorce rate continues, we must realize the need to lend support to the American family. Indeed, education for both boys and girls, starting at the preschool level, needs to be redesigned so that attitudes are not set in the same old mold—attitudes that appear to divide more than to unite.

The groups I developed met in the 70s. Since then, the medical management of birth has changed in several directions. On one side, technology has developed further, to my dismay, and the use of techniques such as fetal monitoring and sonography has become routine. Intervention is also widespread, with the use of spinal blocks, pitocin, epidurals and drugs during labor and delivery. This trend is disturbing because we know a drugged delivery is deleterious for the baby in many ways. One consequence is that the newborn is in the care of doctors and nurses instead of bonding with its mother immediately after birth.

Fortunately, on the other side the art of midwifery has been revived once again and has begun to play an honored role in American obstetrical practice—both in the hospital and at home births. And in many places women are given the freedom to birth in squatting positions or other more natural positions, allowing them to deliver their babies rather than "to be delivered." Also, home births have become an alternative for some. Consumer pressure has been responsible for making alternative choices available, but more pressure is needed to insure good alternatives throughout the country and among all groups of people. Our national health system lends little support to the cause.

However, while attitudes about midwives and the involvement of fathers and the uses of medical technology may have changed, the needs of pregnant couples haven't. One of the tasks is learning to identify conflicts that are primal and personal in comparison to those that are more superficial and culturally influenced. Different types of conflicts call for different solutions. As a society, we need to listen and be responsive to the needs of parents-to-be in order to ensure the emotional and physical well-being of future generations. It is in our own cultural self-interest.

In some cases, changes in the medical system may be necessary; in others, providing ways for couples to turn inward and explore their own past and present will be the solution. To consider, for example, whether they want to have children at all. For many couples, a group may serve as a guiding thread to the way out of the maze. It is one of the important components in the creation of a supportive *environment* of birth—for conception, gestation, and birth and the post-natal period. In fact, evolutionary biologists are now attributing to the role of parenting a more important survival role in their long-term biological view of human behavior, believing there must exist a biochemical base to initiate the parenting behavior so crucial to human survival.

Much has happened in the past decades to make us more aware of childbirth. The deepening of consciousness that began in the 60s and the integration of that awareness into action-oriented programs of the 70s and 80s have been partly responsible. In 1970 when I started in this field, there was much ferment in the area of pregnancy and birth. The resurgence of interest in home births, in both rural and urban areas, fueled by a need by families to regain control of their births, deeply influenced attitudes among parents and health care professionals around the country. The California lay midwifery movement of the 60s was on the cutting edge, challenging parental thinking and the health care system. Midwives and parents spoke out about the shortcomings and risks of routinely technological and clinical birth practices developed during the 40s and 50s. Like many groups in that revolutionary period, these courageous and creative women and the families they served focused a spotlight on an important aspect of our cultural patterning. The births were ritual occasions celebrated lovingly with extended family. The lay midwives' and parent groups' advocacy for women's and babies' rights was in tune with the burgeoning feminist movement of the time. Like any other swing of the pendulum, it became political. Ultimately, their action created change and helped foster a revival of a vital midwifery practice. Although these groups were forced to struggle for authority and respect, the influence of their thinking and action was widely felt. As a result prospective parents were empowered to demand better alternatives to the increasingly mechanistic hospital delivery of their babies.

The escalating cost of a traditional hospital delivery created changes, also, and many young doctors and nurses in obstetrics and family practice took on the challenge of altering the situation. Yet with a declining birth rate, doctors and hospitals wanted to attract expectant parents to their institutions and have altered practices to meet consumer demands.

In the wake of the "consciousness revolution" of the 60s, many "alternative" birth centers were started. The 70s provided us with many models. For example, Mt. Zion Hospital in San Francisco, and other hospitals across the country, introduced a home-like "alternative birth suite" with a minimum of medical equipment and an attractive birthing room that resembled one's own bedroom. New research on the effects of drugs used during delivery and other interventions was taken into account. A most important element in this environment was the quality, tenderness and supportiveness of the medical staff and the commitment of the nurses and nurse-midwives. These changes occurred at Mt. Zion after Dr. Roberta Ballard, the Chief of Pediatrics, experienced what she felt was insensitive treatment during her own labor and delivery at the hospital. Feeling it as an inhumane and threatening environment, she took the lead in establishing a completely new birthing unit.

Studies done by Klaus and Kennell on the importance of mother-child bonding have affected physicians' thinking and altered hospital practice to some extent, and Leboyer's ideas and practices in the 70s influenced parents and some doctors.

Other models of alternative birth environments emerged and faltered due to lack of financial support, AMA blockage, insurance impediments. What has followed is the "alternative birth suite" in many hospitals across the country, a new choice more suited to the needs of the hospitals and its institutional problems. Labor rooms are being converted into Labor/Delivery/ Recovery rooms called LDRs. In this plan, there is but one move after delivery to a Post-Partum room. Alternatively, low-risk patients are offered a room in which labor, delivery and post-partum recovery can all take place. This arrangement seems to satisfy many of the needs of parents and staff. In some few hospitals the use of electronic fetal monitoring (EFM) is limited; in most it is on the increase. In California, its use appears standard—a hundred percent. In some cases, there is more encouragement for the mother in labor to move around (to ambulate) during the first stages of labor. In some hospital settings there is less intrusive intervention, in others *more*. Often the threat of malpractice suits for both physicians and nurses underlies their procedures. But the need to control is evident in most places.

Some freestanding centers (which are not within the hospital itself, but only 7-10 minutes from a back-up hospital) are fortunate enough to have financial support in their home states, like the birth center midwife Elizabeth Gilmore and her colleagues started in Taos, New Mexico in 1980. It still serves the parents of a large rural area. In Menlo Park a limited capacity out-of-hospital center called The Birth Place, initiated through the efforts of Suzanne Arms, author of *The Immaculate Deception,* obstetrician Dr. Don Creevy and others, was opened in the fall of 1979. The ultimate goal was to provide a research center—a full range of alternative birth practices and support services to the community. It survives today although it has become more traditional in its practice. More reliance is placed on nurses than on midwives. It still serves as a model for other communities on the west coast.

Individuals and groups in other parts of the country have also been working toward these changes for a long time. Pioneering efforts date from the turn of the century; for example, the work of the Chicago Maternity Center in the early 1900s, the Frontier Nursing Service in Kentucky in the 1920s, the Maternity Center Association in New York City in the 1940s, all working for natural childbirth, the practice of midwifery and home deliveries. It was at the Maternity Center that I prepared for the births of my three children in the 1950s. I delivered my three children at two of only three hospitals (Columbia Presbyterian and French Hospital in New York City) that then offered "natural childbirth and rooming-in"—an arrangement that allowed my newborn baby to stay with me in my room and allowed my husband to be with his new baby as well.

Back in the 1940s the Maternity Center was training nurse-midwives in New York City and was the first to introduce Dr. Grantley Dick-Read's ideas and methods to the United States. Read was a British obstetrician who in 1942 published a ground-breaking book called *Childbirth Without Fear*. Translated into ten languages, it is still read today.

When almost all women were being delivered under deep anesthesia, he developed a method for "natural childbirth," considering childbearing to be a organic part of the life flow. He began to educate mothers for birth—and fathers as well. It was his contention that fear caused tension and tension caused pain and good preparation was the way to alleviate it. He emphasized both the physiological and psychological aspects by explaining to mothers what was happening in their bodies, by teaching them body and breathing exercises to aid them in the *work* of labor, and by stressing the need for emotional support from fathers and doctors and nurses. He also believed birth was a sacred experience.

That was back in the 1920s. When he toured the United States in the late 1950s, he was impressed by the luxury of American hospitals, but was shocked by the many interventions women were subjected to in the course of normal delivery: the casual use of anesthesia, analgesia and forceps. He spoke of a general servitude toward mechanization and trend toward drugs, shots, syringes, and steely instruments. However, even more upsetting to him was the overuse of oxygen for the newborn baby, whom he said should have been given instead the warmth and security of its mother's breast. He questioned why American women needed so much more specialized medical attention than women all over the world and yet received so little real emotional support.

A sensitive, innovative man—well ahead of his time; holistic and spiritual in nature, drawing on the interdisciplinary wisdom of psychology, sociology, anthropology, history and medicine, he strove for the treatment of the whole person and for the integration of the family during the entire childbearing time. Extremely sensitive to human relationships and metaphysics, he continued throughout his life to work towards an understanding of the underlying laws of nature. A very special obstetrician, he was much misunderstood in his time. Perhaps his anti-establishment views, his spiritual values and his humanism were too "unscientific" for his traditional colleagues.

His book prepared me to move through the experience in a natural way. I guess I didn't need much convincing. I wanted to continue actively participating in the process I'd been involved in for nine months. I certainly didn't want to miss the magical moment of birth. I wanted to be awake! I never regretted my choice, although my first labor was long and arduous and was preceeded by five days of intermittent false labor. Then, as now, I felt strongly about the importance of the symbiosis. I had been my baby's environment for nine formative months, affecting it with my every thought and action. It was important to me therefore, *how* the baby would be born—both the journey and the separation.

The experience was fantastic, and after the birth I was euphoric. In Abraham Maslow's terms it was a "peak experience." The euphoria *had* to be shared as a family. Having us all together in my room for the hours after birth was immensely important for me and, I believe, for all of us.

I remember the births of my three children as incredible experiences; the discomfort of labor—even the pain—was quickly erased by the post-birth jubilation, and what remains is my positive attitude about childbirth. The positivity surprises me now, as it did years ago. I could never figure out how I came by it; certainly not from my conditioning. My mother had a difficult time giving birth, and I doubt that there was much positive folklore about the joy of childbirth in her Czech-Jewish background. I'm sure her forebears labored long and hard delivering their children and passed agonizing tales on to their daughters. My sister and I had heard how difficult and painful my mother's experience had been. My sister went along with the conventions of the day and chose anesthesia. It was a shame because her labors were extremely short. Quite recently, as she and I talked about birth, she recalled her awe at my determination to deliver without anesthesia in the Grantley Dick-Read method of "painless childbirth." She spoke poignantly, for she felt she had deprived herself and her husband of an integrating experience that would have been helpful to their marriage and their relationship with the new baby. All of this seems hardly startling now, as we have incorporated so many of his ideas into our system, and even so, not enough has changed.

Ruth Lubic, long-time director of the Maternity Center, and her colleagues have continued to pioneer new alternatives, and in the 70s opened a clinic for nurse-midwife attended births within seven minutes of a hospital in New York City. They are still at the forefront today. Unfortunately, large prestigious teaching hospitals geared to high-risk births have had a harder time responding to the demand for alternative birthing services within the hospital. The University of California, San Francisco, is one that has met the demand. Recently, I visited their Birth Center and I felt they have responded sensitively to the climate of the time—medically and socially. Their six newly renovated birthing suites for labor and delivery offer some of the most beautiful views in San Francisco. They are large, commodious, rooms fashionably furnished—like rooms at San Francisco's most exclusive hotels. Medical equipment for emergency use is carefully hidden behind doors along one wall. Separate rooms for post-partum use are provided since it is not expedient to tie up the use of the labor rooms. It is well done. As a university teaching hospital, they also serve a wide population, including high-risk medical patients, caring for HIV-positive patients and crack-addicted mothers.

Consumer pressure and the reality of the marketplace have created change in various directions. "Many parents want to do natural childbirth and want more control during labor and delivery," said one New York obstetrician. Dr. Raymond Van de Wiele, head of obstetrics at Columbia Presbyterian Hospital in New York says, "Using a birthing room is good medicine." Doctors now accept the idea that a homelike environment may be healthier for mother and baby and that having fathers and other support people present, including the baby's siblings, can be important to the mother's equanimity, and therefore to the newborn's well-being. In the 1960s ten to fifteen percent of fathers attended the birth of their children. In contrast, by 1982 eighty-five percent did so. A supportive person may be there also or may replace the father.

Newly designed birthing beds are incorporated into the LDR and LDP rooms. Beds that look like residential beds have motor driven, split frame mattresses and are adjustable to various positions during delivery. A laboring mother can labor and deliver in the same room. The birthing rooms create an expectation of normal delivery which affects not only the attitudes of the mother and father or extended family member, but the health professionals involved. In a less clinical, more homelike environment, there seems to be less tendency to speed things up. Also there is much evidence that a woman who is ambulatory during labor has an easier labor. Not all doctors are enthusiastic, however, and many prefer the old labor and delivery rooms. Perhaps old habits and attitudes underlie their positions. Their lack of enthusiasm, on the other hand, may reflect an increasing incidence of litigation if something goes wrong. Many doctors rely on the latest in medical technology in their practice and insist on electronic fetal monitors, intravenous glucose hookups and the use of painkilling drugs, pitocin, and epidural blocks during labor and delivery. Obviously, this equipment and methodology of control is antithetical to natural childbirth and the comfortable self-determining environment of birthing rooms. One of the most alarming trends in the medicalization of birth is the enormous increase in caesarean sections all over the country—from 25% to 50%. It becomes an urgent responsibility for parents to interview potential doctors, to choose those whose ideas and methods about birthing are compatible with their own.

Anne Hubbell Maiden speaks of a wonderful model for a serious international problem. It is called the Village for Mothers and Children in Milan, Italy, in which care for extraordinarily high-risk, homeless, teenage mothers is provided. Their record for delivering healthy babies is outstanding. Young pregnant women become residents early in their pregnancies. They live in small houses with other pregnant women and other mothers and children. In this supportive environment, they learn about pregnancy and mothering, can continue their schooling while they send their children to preschool or can complete job training. They are allowed to stay through pregnancy, birth and the early years of motherhood, in fact, until their child is three. At the time of birth, they are attended by experienced midwives and supported by their friends in the community. What a remarkable solution to an increasingly difficult community problem. Dr. Maiden points to the multiple advantages to mother and child, and to society, as pregnant mothers are given continuous support care during a time of crisis. Emotional and physical health reverse a potentially negative scenario.

Since the 60s, we have witnessed a positive revolution in attitudes toward nature and environment, towards health, and toward the personal management of family birth. It seems that women—and men—want to reown their bodies, minds and feelings. Over lunch with English author and childbirth educator Sheila Kitzinger years ago, I questioned why the alternative birth movement broke through the barriers in the 70s. Kitzinger replied,

> It seems there comes a time when people can hear. The great propagandists are ones who understand timing and don't say more than people can hear at a given moment. It seems extraordinary to me that people are able to now hear the very same words that were being spoken for many long years. In order to present an idea, it has to be bold and simple. I think that's what Leboyer has done by focusing a strong light on one particular area and one defined moment in human experience.

Despite all the new information that has accumulated, and the increased availability of childbirth preparation classes, women who are pregnant for the first time are still as excited *and* as uncertain and anxious, and perhaps less supported, now than women have been since the beginning of time. Women and men still have to discover the complexities of the pregnant state for themselves. They need an environment in which they can take a critical look at the important changes taking place in their lives during the journey into the unknown. This knowledge seems inaccessible on a conscious level before pregnancy and there is little in our educational or societal system to prepare us earlier. Unlike other transitions in our lives, giving birth and becoming parents isn't a passage that we consider very much until its actuality and immediacy is upon us.

Most recently, in reviewing shifts of attitude and practice, I spoke to some of the doctors and midwives whom I had joined in an effort to start a freestanding birth center in Marin County in northern California fifteen years ago. Our year-long process had been halted by lack of funding. Among my former colleagues was Suellen Miller, nurse-midwife and partner in an obstetrical practice in northern California, who reported:

> "Mothers-to-be of the late 80s and 90s are now seeking more control over the experience and, like their mothers of the 50s and early 60s, want pain-free deliveries. There is rejection once again of "natural" childbirth. In choosing to combine careers with motherhood, and having little time to enjoy pregnancy, they are opting for a different selection among the possibilities. They choose not to experience the discomfort of birth—they want the baby but not the process. They want the labor, delivery and postpartum room where their husbands can be present but also prefer epidural blocks and painkilling drugs. Yet they do attend Lamaze classes."

"Expectations change," says Suellen Miller's partner, obstetrician Dr. Ed Boyce of Larkspur, California, who is one of those who pioneered the idea of father involvement in natural childbirth. Not what he would prefer, but a philosophic attitude.

Polyglot as our culture is, we have no rituals around this rite of passage. Left behind in the cities and villages of Europe, Asia, Africa, South America are the customs that guided men and women through this period. What remains is a loosely defined notion of what is masculine and feminine, of how feelings should be dealt with, of how women and babies should be considered. Probably our loss of customs has helped place the medical model in such a powerful position.

Since we no longer have these supportive cultural traditions in place to guide us, there are no traditional ways to cope with the intense emotions that accompany the dramatic psychological changes that occur. We know that unresolved issues, fears and fantasies have an important effect on labor, birth, bonding, and the baby's and family's future. The very existence of these fears indicates the need to deal with the emotional content of pregnancy sensitively, with mutual support groups and psychological counselors and family. Therein lies support for the crisis. Present day swings in attitude indicate this.

In the 1950s Grete Bibring was one of the early articulate advocates in America for the potential usefulness of the psychological support groups that this book advocates. Unfortunately, her ideas, communicated to other professionals in the late 1950s, have still not become part of routine prenatal care. Others, like Sheila Kitzinger, English anthropologist, author and childbirth educator, have advocated these ideas since then, as has Niles Newton in the United States, and many others. Based on my own experience with pregnant couples in the support groups I have led, I know there is an urgent need for such workshops, as a complement to the recent resurgence of interest in making delivery more natural for mother and child and the family, and as an antidote to the swing backward to the preference for drugs during delivery. As early as 1959, Bibring pointed out our tendency to overemphasize the obstetrical aspects of pregnancy and birth. The warning still applies. According to Bibring:

> Pregnancy, like puberty or menopause, is a period of crisis involving profound psychological as well as somatic change. As the modern family becomes isolated, and as other important group memberships break down, the individual must rely increasingly on the nuclear family, especially on the marital relationship, and this unit is rarely equipped to replace all these figures in their varied supportive functions.

> With increasing emphasis on the "scientific" in our society, less and less attention is paid to the unscientific, the irrational, the emotional and spiritual dimensions of human existence. We see often exaggerated attempts on the part of the expectant mother to adjust consciously to the scientific viewpoints of pregnancy and its management.

We may have to direct our attention to the period of pregnancy itself and find adequate ways to bring the psychological support in line with the achievements of today's
obstetrics.

"Some Considerations of the Psychological
Processes in Pregnancy", Grete L. Bibring,

How each parent deals with this rite of passage depends not
only on his or her unique personal history, but also on our
shared socio-cultural history. Actually, the physical care and psychological nurturance of pregnant parents and thereby of the
baby developing in the womb is the social responsibility of society. A wise prenatal health program needs support and funding
by the government and the private sector. Indeed, we have a
responsibility to the next generation.

In a recent report of a Public Health Service Expert Panel,
"Caring For Our Future: The Content of Prenatal Care issued in
1989 by the U.S. Government Department of Health and Human
Services, there is a careful and thorough assessment of the needs
of the pregnant period for the mother, child and family. There
was agreement that the psychosocial aspects of pregnancy were
in serious need of investigation. It is obviously imperative for us
to focus on how we manage this period of life as a society, as
we read of increasing incidence of child abuse, HIV-positive
babies, crack babies, alcoholic babies. Neglect of these issues is
very costly to us all. For example, one dollar spent on early and
continuous prenatal care is juxtaposed against three dollars for
repair and continued care of later post-birth problems. The lack
of prenatal education and care is often the cause of high-risk
births—and consequently of premature and low-weight babies at
birth.

As a society we cannot afford these results. Man, woman and
child—each one of us is deeply involved in this experience of
coming into being and birth. We come at it every which way—
scientifically, intuitively, socially, spiritually, mystically. The way
we view it affects the way we manage the process, the way we
behave, the way the baby will develop in the womb. The creation of holistic family-centered environments for birth—birth

centers that incorporate old ideas and new ones, weaving together the strands of intuition and knowledge and experience—are an important next step.

A Holistic Family Birth Center

When I visited many years ago with A.S. Neill, author of *Summerhill* and headmaster of an innovative nontraditional English school, he related a story about one of the small children in his school who, in a fight with a classmate, hurt his hand rather badly. When the school nurse examined it, she decided that it required hospital care. As she set out to drive the boy to the local hospital, he insisted on seeing Neill first. "What can I do for you that the nurse can't do?" asked Neill of the teary boy, who insisted that Neill drive him to the hospital. The small boy looked up at the six-foot-tall Scotsman with love and trust and said, "She'll take care of my hand, but you'll take care of all of me."

This same attitude is the concept of holistic medicine. It is an approach to health that considers the whole person, not only his/her illness or problem, but the integration of mind, body, spirit. It is a view of the person in relation to the entire context of his life—the family, work, social and cultural milieu, the environment. Viewing a person from a standpoint of health and normal stressful transition in the life cycle rather than illness and trauma, encourages participation in the healing process in an active and informed way. Holistic approaches include many nontraditional healing practices such as acupuncture, meditation and visualization, exercise, nutrition. All have been ignored in Western medicine until recently.

A thousand years ago, the Chinese organized prenatal clinics to guide a woman through pregnancy, believing that her emotions and biology together influenced the nature and future behavior and mental health of her child. It was called *Tai-kyo*—"embryonic education." They believed a happy, healthy mother produced a happy, healthy child. Consequently, the culture fostered emotional tranquility as well as physical well-being. We, too, need places that are concerned not only with our bodies, but also with our psyches and spirit.

We need to create holistic environments in which expectant parents are physically cared for and psychologically supported during this important rite of passage—environments that help them practice life as an art while involved with the very essence of being: the creation of a new person. We need to provide opportunities for them to explore ways to loosen the psychological knots, to reassess and reorient their lives as they prepare for parenthood—environments in which they begin to understand what governs their choices. Professionals can guide them into developing their own inner resources, allowing parents to rise to the pleasures and responsibilities of their new state in their own individual ways. Birth centers would enable expectant parents to celebrate the transformation taking place instead of "laboring" through the transition. We need environments in which everything important about birth could be discussed, evaluated and acted on during the childbearing year.

Many questions need to be raised by parents, health professionals, social scientists, foundations distributing funds, insurance companies, government agencies, medical associations—all those involved in the delivery and regulation of health care needed by expectant parents.

What could a modern birth center offer a couple both before and after they conceive? Imagine that parents were able to come to the center before conception simply to consider whether or not they wanted to have a baby. Imagine that they had others to talk with as they worked through their ambivalent feelings about becoming parents—others who might be skilled counselors or parents who were further along on the parenting journey—just as Alan and Rachael did. In this environment, they might have an opportunity to cuddle a friend's drowsy, sweet-smelling infant or try to quiet a wet, cranky toddler as they all talked, just as young people used to and probably still do in smaller, more intimate communities where life is simpler and families and friends are closer and more involved in each other's lives. It might enable them to plan with more emotional clarity and spiritual empowerment. By loosening the psyche's knots even before conception, they might be able to resolve their ambivalence and be able to participate more fully in the parental experience. They might bring to the creative moment of conception a level of radiant consciousness and deep love that would transfer to the person coming into being. How different is the act of creation when a child is conceived out of love and is invited, as it were, to come into being? How might the atmosphere of love be felt by the developing organism? We know that stress is communicated to the baby—why not joy and love?

During "the pregnant year" the birth center would serve all stages of preconception, pregnancy, birth and the first few postpartum months, giving support to the emergent family as it progresses through its growing pains. The three-generational family, any unit of mother and child and significant others, or any family configuration, would be included as well, for we know that this passage affects siblings, grandparents and extended families directly and indirectly in important ways. So far removed are we these days from an integrated view of family life that we tend to overlook the impact on all involved.

A birth center could provide an environment where there is continuity of experience with other expectant parents and with a professional staff of doctors, nurse-midwives, psychologists, and childbirth educators, who serve as knowledgeable guides throughout the entire period. Experienced, well-trained nurse-midwives are important to the concept of the birth center. Traditionally throughout history, experienced women trained in midwifery have guided other women through pregnancy and birth. Starting in early pregnancy they can provide warm, supportive, compassionate attention and medical care. During labor and birth, their continuous attendance maintains a familiar and feminine supportive presence as they try not to disturb the mother's own natural way of giving birth. Dr. Michel Odent, after many years of delivering babies and also observing the midwives at the maternity clinic, speaks of the appropriateness of "authentic" midwives attending birthing mothers. He feels "birth becomes easier, less painful, shorter and less dangerous." He also feels the presence of a male doctor can often be inhibiting.

"Midwives," says Suellen Miller, "allow the mother to become the heroine, as Joseph Campbell describes the heroine's journey, moving through the transformation feeling as if it is she, herself, who is doing this wonderful, amazing thing—giving birth. As a nurse-midwife, I am, of course, in favor of midwives. But I am also the partner of a wonderful obstetrician, Ed Boyce. As we work together, I see how sensitive, tender and patient he is. His sensitivity is like that of a midwife. He respects how the birthing process works and the way women's bodies work. He's understanding and allows time, waiting for the process to unfold. He counsels wisely and presents the options."

A trained staff can be sensitive to the emotional well-being of the couple, as well as to the physical aspects of giving birth. The holistic birth center can be a place where people communicate with the heart as well as with the intellect, where the unborn child can experience harmony, where parents can practice listening to their own innate wisdom and can honor their extraordinary state of consciousness. The parents and their health team can meet and come to know one another as they embark on this journey. Together, they can reach personal decisions that reflect their values and life design rather than having to fit into institutionalized choices, methods and routines. Parents can thereby participate in their own evolution and in the evolution of the center as well.

It can be an environment in which parents learn about their bodies and psyches, a place in which they can share the responsibility for their own inner development, health and well-being and participate in their own care. Obviously, no one wants to ignore the benefits of modern medicine. However, it is inappropriate to treat normal pregnancy as an illness. Ninety-five percent of all births are low risk. Birth centers do not mock medical advances or circumvent them; rather, they make use of increased scientific knowledge to enhance the experience, not to control it. It is important psychologically to disassociate the normal process of birthing from the environment of a hospital, which is designed for the sick. It is also important that the ambience of the center projects a sense of order and strives to reduce uncertainty, to engender feelings of familiarity and security, to be enfolding and tranquil. It can be a place in which parents may create new personal rituals out of shared experience.

The practical plan for services at the center might be divided into four stages—preconception, pregnancy, delivery and post-natal—each characterized by both unique and interrelated concerns. At each stage, three levels of the experience would be considered: intrapersonal (our relationship to ourselves), interpersonal (relationship with others), and transpersonal (the relationship beyond the boundaries of our own ego-selves—the universal dimension).

The center would be designed to reflect the symbolic and specific aspects of the lives of the individuals in the group it serves. In some cultures, these important passages are celebrated with supportive others in attendance; in others, quite privately. It is important to honor these roots. We know that unconscious levels of the psyche are activated during this period. In fact, it may be one of the most significant aspects of the experience that leads to further growth.

One of the most relevant arguments for home birth is the familiarity of the setting. This same argument can apply to a well-conceived birth center. At home, all the subtle patterns are comfortable, known, secure. There need be no unconscious search for recognizable symbols; they have been chosen and accepted and are part of the fabric of one's daily existence. When so much change is taking place, having to deal with unfamiliar people, and physical space, and institutional rules adds stress. A physician friend said, "Putting a couple in a strange hospital room and asking the woman to give birth is like asking a couple to make love while we watch." A birth center can be an atmosphere that has already become incorporated into one's psyche as a known and familiar environment, a source of comfort and support.

Each environment has a message. Its voice is as clear as the verbal message of the person who receives the parents as they enter the center. Parents, in their uniquely vulnerable state, will be as sensitive to that message as photographic paper is when exposed to light.

In a warm enveloping physical setting, staffed with affirming, knowing guides—teachers, doctors, nurse-midwives, psychologists and others—we can offer prenatal education and care, films, lectures, and workshops.

Heterogeneous groups of couples and single parents at different stages of pregnancy would explore together their everyday feelings along with the extraordinary and the less-examined psycho-social aspects of pregnancy. They would be able to focus on all aspects of the developing relationship of the mother and the father and the unborn child in an atmosphere of increasing intimacy and trust, comforted by loving others bearing witness to this important event.

Professionals agree that women who receive prenatal care during the first trimester have better pregnancy outcomes than women who have little or no prenatal care. Providing emotional support for both mother- and father-to-be increases their ease in moving through the pregnancy and birth into parenting. They will enjoy a better quality of life, as will their child.

What would be available to a couple at the center? The birth center would be a facility for preconception counseling, prenatal care, labor, delivery and birthing, and postnatal care. It would serve those who can expect a normal, uncomplicated pregnancy and birth—low-risk births, as hospitals call them. This group represents the largest percentage of women giving birth. Preventive care and early detection of existing or potential problems would be a valuable part of the program. Proper screening must take place, of course, to make sure that all mothers-to-be are indeed low-risk! Emergency arrangements would be available for unforeseen problems at the time of labor and delivery, both at the center and at a backup hospital situated no more than seven to ten minutes away. The following section suggests some of the attributes of an ideal birth center.

Psychological (Counseling)

- Counseling with professionals

- Self-led groups

- Preconception groups

- Pregnancy groups

- Individual and couple therapy with professionals

- Postnatal groups

- Infant psychology Early childhood family groups (up to the time the child can speak of its prebirth and birth experience)

Physiological (Medical)

- Prenatal education, care, checkups

- Videos and information about prenatal development and mother's developmental stages

- Nutritional and exercise information and classes

- Midwife consultation—physician consultation

- Prepared childbirth techniques—methods of all kinds

- Preparation for parenting—breastfeeding information and physical aspects of infant care

Physical Space (Environment)

- Reception room with welcoming symbolic entry

- Kitchen for waiting, meeting, gathering, eating, sharing, "kitchen table therapy"

- Garden for conversing, sitting contemplatively, strolling, planting, waiting

- Meeting rooms for group sessions, mind-body practices, yoga, meditation, biofeedback, breathing practices, massage, water therapy

- Staff room

- Music room for listening, making music

- Reference library—books, records, tapes, films, periodicals

- Seminar rooms for teaching midwives, nurses, doctors, for sharing concepts with visitors

- Thrift shop for maternity and infant clothes and children's furniture

- Examination rooms and bathrooms

- Clinical lab

- Emergency rooms

- Three to six birthing rooms reached by a separate entrance through the garden—double beds, extra bed for partner or coach (using the newest experience of teaching hospitals)

- Rooms for midwives and obstetricians to retire and rest, to be on call

To facilitate the process of "loosening the knots," many ways of exploring consciousness developed in Eastern philosophy and by the human potential development movement can be used, techniques like Gestalt, psychodrama, transactional analysis; body techniques involving movement, sound and massage; methods of meditation, psychosynthesis and dream therapies. Journal-keeping can be encouraged as a creative way of recording poems and drawings and of understanding dreams and fantasies during this evocative period

Various techniques would be taught to ease the tension and pain that may develop during labor and delivery, to obviate the need for pain-killing drugs, including meditation, hypnosis, biofeedback training, breath control techniques like those of hatha yoga and kundalini yoga, sound anesthesia like chants, mantras and music. Also available can be the methods taught by Lamaze, Odent, Kitzinger, Bradley, and others. But most of all, emphasis would be on confirming women's own intuitive wisdom.

Imagine a center either in the city, overlooking a park, or outside the center of the city, close to the healing effects of water, to the woods or mountains and yet within minutes of a hospital. Whether in the city, the suburbs, or the country, it would be a space flooded with natural light so essential to growing things. Imagine an airy pavilion of loosely connected rooms surrounding a garden, the entrance door reached through a passage covered with a bower of flowering vines. Imagine this rite of passage symbolically expressed in the design of the entrance gate—the way in and out—a metaphor so particular to conception and birth. If, as Carl Jung suggests, the house is the symbol of the self beyond the body, the need for the birth house is a metaphoric expression of this transformation in spatial form. The place, the physical space, is designed to be a calm, secure, protective, enveloping environment—a symbolic womb for parents-to-be as they cross the threshold into parenthood. It is an environment designed to receive a new spirit transiting from one state of existence to another, says Marc Olivier in *The Psychology of the House*.

> Every threshold crossed marks a new state, every door entered a step forward in constant renewal, where the wheel of life expands and contracts, following the universal spiral, leading humanity from inside to outside, from periphery to center, in a rhythm inexorably tied to that of the planets and the atom.

As one moves across the threshold and through the portal, there is a welcoming central reception room which in turn opens into a garden seen through glassy walls.

The garden is central to the plan. In it I envision a large tree with low, spreading limbs—a tree of life, an elemental symbol in all cultures. A tree to sit in and under—an enveloping organic reminder of the changing seasons and the processes of regeneration and birth.

I see the garden filled with life—abounding with the colors, smells, sounds, rhythms and movement of living things: birds, small animals, flowering plants, moving water, fertile earth. Water is part of the ritual of birth in many cultures—and is used in healing. It connects us symbolically to our own beginnings. The care and growth of the garden would reflect and affirm a similar process taking place for the parents as the pregnancy unfolds. It would have the simplicity and tranquility of a Japanese garden, reiterating the elements of the universe, with its rocks, water, trees, earth, sky.

In many cultures, a tree-planting ceremony has been customary after a birth: in Switzerland, it is an apple tree for a boy, a pear tree for a girl; in Haiti, a coconut tree for both. Recently, some young friends of mine in Massachusetts created such a ceremony after the birth of their first child. The mother happened to be an anthropologist:

> For Peter, who was born three days ago: We buried your placenta and planted a tree above it to represent your connection with the earth and all of life. Next to it, we buried a peach, an apple and a plum, symbolizing you, the fruit of my womb and the seed of our lives.

Parents might create their own personal tree planting ceremony. Can you imagine a more beautiful way to reforest the earth?

The garden can serve as a place to talk with others, to read, or simply to be alone in contemplative silence—a place to sense one's own rhythms and those of mother and child and the rhythm of the universe to which each of us is attuned.

Woven into the fabrics of the furnishings and decorating the walls would be birth images from all over the world to nourish our intuitive understanding of the designs and artifacts that symbolize the universal mystery, magic and miracle of birth—

symbols that protect and inspire subliminal confidence, and represent women as they move through this rite of passage. Photos and art would emanate a feeling of the Goddess. Every birthing mother wants to be treated like a Queen, a Goddess.

Homelike rooms, large enough to accommodate family or friends, would ideally have a deep bathtub/shower, toilet and a washbasin. It would be wonderful to plan rooms that opened onto balconies overlooking the garden.

Creating furnishings for the center might be part of the activity of the workshops: weaving or painting or working together with birth symbols on a wall hanging reminiscent of the old-fashioned quilting parties. Fathers might make furniture for the center and for their babies. Textures of wool, straw, reed and pottery would mirror the organic nature of the gestation and birth process. Particular consideration would be given to the healing qualities of water, color, sound and light, and the tactile sense of materials—the psychological effects of the sensory environment. For example, sound is used in various cultures during labor and delivery: music by the Laotians of Southeast Asia, the Navajo Indians and the Cuna Indians of Panama; and conversation as sound stimulation to ease birth pain by many tribes who pattern delivery as a social event. Sontag's research, among other research, demonstrates that sound affects both the mother and the unborn child. We would benefit from the use of research into the healing and soothing qualities of sound.

Earth colors might prevail: warm embracing combinations of golden yellows, pomegranate reds, persimmon oranges accented by indigo and sky-blues, plum-purples and the leaf-greens of springtime: reds, yellows, oranges used to excite, delight and stimulate; blues and greens to soothe and comfort. There is a science of color to draw upon and a designer's intuitive sense to engage.

Comfortable chairs and couches would enfold one, keeping in mind the needs of the pregnant body. Flexible seating arrangements can invite all kinds of exchange in both group and private consultation and can promote informal conversation and friendship. Close by the sitting room, a large kitchen can provide a family atmosphere in which people might gather at a circular wooden table for food or hot drinks near a warming fire. In this nurturing environment, food, feelings, knowledge and experience can be shared, and extended family support systems can develop quite naturally. Kitchen table consultation can take place informally with staff about everything from nutrition and treatment of simple ailments to demands of the emerging family. Exchange about the most intimate and urgent concerns might take place among the parents quite casually over tea.

Other rooms that serve particular functions can surround the atrium. Consultation and examining rooms, designed in a warm, nonclinical fashion, would contain the necessary medical and technical equipment and would encourage trusting, self-responsible interactions between staff and clients. Rooms for group meetings and for various body therapies can be available for healthy exercise, pleasure and sensory expansion: spaces for group work, for dancing, for yoga, for meditation, for massage, saunas and mineral baths. New aids, such as biofeedback training, found to be helpful for relaxation and for teaching about one's inner states would also be available, as would a library filled with the newest books, periodicals, records, films, cassettes, slides about childbirth and parenting, self-care and self-awareness, and a music room for listening to and making music.

Lighting in the rooms would be controlled by dimmers, allowing parents and medical staff to select the level of light they prefer during labor. Chairs and beds designed for comfort and flexibility and facilitation of labor and delivery would furnish rooms in which double beds would accommodate fathers and mothers and perhaps small children in the family, or midwives. Parents would bring personal belongings: musical instruments or tapes so that they can play music, games or pieces of art to meditate on—whatever gives comfort and feels more like home, just as the couple in my group did:

> We took a lot of things from home like a book of poetry, a quilt (which we never used but it made us feel good to have it folded on a chair and available) and favorite records.

Inspiration for architectural designs can come from the shapes of the earliest dwellings of man, such as caves, shelters that reiterate womb shapes. We might choose circular dwellings such as are used by many societies that live in close harmony with their natural environment: the igloos of the Eskimos, the wigwams of the Indians, the *kraals* of the African tribes and the *yurts* of the Mongols, the contemporary geodesic dome of Buckminster Fuller, or the sculptured shapes of Paoli Soleri in Arizona, which also invite the interaction of man and nature. Or spaces might be inspired by the shapes that the animal world uses to build its nests, cocoons and shelters. The spherical configuration of a dome attunes us to the celestial environment, to the rising and setting sun, to the phases of the moon, solstices and equinoxes. Imagine giving birth under the stars and the light of the full moon. Many births occur at the time of the full moon. Imagine a dome that unfolds like a lotus, opening to the warm breezes of the spring, summer or fall sky.

The aperture, "the eye of the dome," as Mircea Eliade puts it, "has classically symbolized breakthrough from plane to plane, communication with the transcendent." Childbirth itself is such an opening. "There are forms derived from the study of sacred architecture that we can use," says Ken Mackenzie, architect-designer who employs the principles of sacred geometry in his work, "forms derived from the circle—domes, rounds, curved walls that are representative of the heavenly realm. Ancient knowledge which dealt with number and proportion, musical harmony, color and geometry is being studied and utilized anew. We can once again design in harmony with the universal order, realigning the body on all levels and creating health, vitality and well-being."

This dream of childbearing opens up the possibilities of an alternate reality for the pregnant year. I am reminded of the teaching of the Senoi tribe in Malaysia, who ask their children when they have a nightmare to sleep again and re-create a less frightening scenario in order to repattern their behavior and experience. Similarly, there is creative potential in a positive dream of childbirth. Let us create a vision of the possible.

Pregnancy is an incredibly dynamic period for all involved. The baby developing in its complex container is integrally linked to its parents and to the unique texture of their lives and to the outer environment. Everyone involved is integrally connected to the wonder, the potential, and the miracle of the life process. The more we are aware, the more wondrous it becomes. Let us create an environment for the pregnant year and birth that reflects the glory and mystery of being human—a harmonious environment in which a sense of serenity can be transmitted to the person growing in the womb. Let us celebrate birth and honor it in a uniquely individual way.

Giving birth can be a deeply intimate and expansive experience for both partners. Even as it is grounded in one of the most basic and repeatable of human experiences, it can be a window to the intrinsic patterns of the universe and to the archetypal cycles of life and death that have existed since the first matter crossed that indefinable boundary line and took the form of living cells.

APPENDIX:
EXERCISES FOR EXPLORING THE
EMOTIONS OF PREGNANCY

Exercises do not do anything in themselves; they merely help to focus attention and awareness, a little like a microscope magnifying the field it examines in detail. They can be tools that allow you to move beneath your usual guises and defensive layers to deeper levels of intuition.

Just as dreams open a window for you to observe the complex strands of personal behavior patterns, so can these exercises. They enable you to practice new skills in order to change behavior, once outmoded patterns are recognized. It's a little like learning a new dance. First, you watch how it's done, then you start to practice moving your body differently so that you can do the new steps. Once you can handle the movements skillfully, you no longer need to focus on the individual steps and you find yourself dancing, freely and unselfconsciously.

Years of creative exploration and testing have created a wealth of material to draw on. Many of these methods have grown over the past twenty years out of the fields of humanistic and transpersonal psychology. The exercises that follow are gleaned from my years of personal experience as a group member and leader. Others I improvised as the need for them arose. I am particularly proud of the ones I originated, Dialoging with the unborn, Listening to the child within, and The Gift, among others, that have now found their ways into other's work and are used widely. Still others may be found in the growing literature on alternative techniques for enhancing personal growth and self-knowledge. I have listed some that I have found useful (see Bibliography).

The needs and patterns of individuals and groups will vary.

Some groups may be more verbal and need methods that develop their weaker skills, such as nonverbal communication; others may already be comfortable with nonverbal ways of communicating and will need to practice articulating their feelings more clearly. In my experience, a structured exercise is often very helpful in understanding unexplained moods or behavior patterns and revealing deeper layers of feelings that are provoking specific behavior.

Some of the people in my groups felt exercises weren't necessary, that simply talking together was as effective in working through problems. Others loved them. One man, in particular, felt that talking to his unborn child while it was still in the womb was a profound and moving experience that affected the development of their relationship later on. That probably is true. Personally, I feel these methods cut through carefully guarded defenses more quickly since we're all so skillful at using words to cover our real feelings!

Sadly, most of us have not been rewarded for showing our true feelings, especially men, and have consequently learned to hide them. Most of us have learned all too well. We try to suppress our feelings, which has a crippling effect on our lives. We are lost without the information they provide. Our emotions and feelings are checkpoints for our sense of balance and equilibrium as we respond to the world around us. Through emotion we sense our feelings of anger, frustration, joy, love, peace. If our hearts are closed, deep experience does not touch us. Give life to your emotions.

The exercises that follow are some that may be used for either group sessions, with two couples, or individually. If you plan to use them on your own at home, I might suggest that you have your partner or a friend whose voice you like make an audiotape for you of various exercises. Then you can lie down quietly and listen at leisure when you are in the mood. Ask the reader to speak slowly, allowing enough time for you to follow the directions without feeling rushed or having to strain to keep up. The point of these exercises is to move into quiet inner places. Be sure to find a relaxed time when you will not be interrupted. Dim the lights. Spend a few silent moments lying down before you even turn on the tape. Create the same time and space and peaceful ambience for yourself as you would for others. Start to learn how to be a good parent to yourself. Try to set aside time each day or at least three times a week.

These exercises are simply a stimulant—a guide to creating your own designs, perhaps, for you know better than anyone what you need. Don't feel that there is anything sacred about these suggestions. Although there is experience behind them, it is important that they be personally meaningful. So, feel free to adapt them to your own images and symbols. I want to emphasize that there is no routine way to design these groups and that this is not an infallible recipe book. Other methods may be gathered from the books listed in the Bibliography.

Follow your feelings and your intuition and be responsive to the needs of the group members.

Remember, too, feelings are neither good nor bad. Don't prejudge your feelings and clam up.

Becoming aware of what you are feeling, and beyond that, what you need can open up communication between you and your partner. The more conscious you become, the more insight you have about yourself, and the more you have to share will enrich your relationships with others. You will feel more in charge of your life. You will probably also receive more affection, understanding and love.

BREATHING AND RELAXATION EXERCISES

The source of our existence is our breath—breathing in and breathing out. From our earliest time in the womb environment, a steady, uninterrupted flow of oxygen is crucial to our existence. Once born, each breath we draw initiates a miraculous set of complex occurrences which cleanse, oxygenate and feed our entire system. We are dependent on each breath, each inhalation and exhalation. The way we choose to breathe in turn affects our way of being—our physical and emotional tone and health. Even though this may seem obvious, we need to remind ourselves of its essential function in our lives. It seems particularly important during pregnancy and labor to be at ease with one's breathing, to understand its function in relaxing tension, in being attuned to the baby and one's partner, in letting go, in maintaining balance.

Try to do a relaxation exercise before each exercise at home, or at the beginning of the evening in the group.

Many people control their feelings through their breathing pattern, often with shallow breathing or quick short breaths. I remember when I was little and scared, I controlled my fear by holding my breath. I still do unconsciously. If instead, I take deep, long slow breaths, wondrous things occur. My heart rate will drop twenty or twenty-five beats a minute, as will my blood pressure. As the body relaxes, the nervous system quiets. Energy begins to flow and there is a sensation of motion and emotion that may be expressed in crying or laughing or anger and in physical action provoked by the feelings that surface.

Becoming aware of our breathing patterns and habits helps us see how we take in the world around us and how we let it go. For centuries, the Yoga schools of different traditions in the East have taught breathing awareness exercises in order to relax, to quiet the chatter of thoughts (the monkey mind, the Buddhists call it), and to achieve balance of mind, body, and spirit. These practices can help us to become attuned to the larger universal rhythm of which we are so integrally a part.

Spending some time alone (or with a partner) doing these breathing exercises is a positive way to initiate the sensitive attunement that will be required during pregnancy and labor and in the development of family life with your baby.

EXERCISE 1: FIRST WARM-UP

This exercise is a good one to start off the evening, helpful in making the transition from the work day.

Lie down on the floor. Close your eyes and get as comfortable as you can, and, for a few breaths, concentrate on the air going in and out. Notice that you relax more as you breathe out and that there is a slight tension as you breathe in. Notice at the end of expiration there is a brief moment when the chest stops moving completely before it takes another breath. This is the moment of deepest relaxation and is our own internal means of momentary relaxation. Try to exaggerate the moment when your breath is all the way out, just before you take in another breath.

Now imagine that your entire body is a vessel for air and not only your lungs but your whole body fills and empties with each breath...Imagine the air filling up your whole body, all the way down to your toes. You can actually begin to feel your whole body breathing and expanding as it takes a breath and then you let go of that breath.

Imagine the breath going all the way down to the toes and that you breathe out through your feet, leaving them relaxed, emptying them of their tension. Concentrate on that end point of breathing, filling your legs each time with the new breath and emptying them out. Now fill your legs up to the thighs, feeling your legs expand and contract. Now let the breath go to your toes, your groin and now the lower back. Feel the muscles soften at the end of each breath...

Now out the chest, the lower abdomen, feel the stomach muscles soften, now the chest itself, filling the whole body with air and letting it all out. No force is necessary. The air can move itself.

Now the shoulders...let them fill and empty. Let them feel soft and droopy. And the arms. Now the neck...let the neck and the rest of your body fill, empty, soften. And your head...feel your head getting lighter and more relaxed...Continue to breathe gently and when you are ready, open your eyes.

Now your arms and hands...You may notice a sensation of flowing as your body fills and then empties. Now your head and scalp and your facial muscles...Notice how heavy your jaw is...Let your face fill with air...For a few breaths, let your whole body fill and empty, the air moving up and down, feel it all over and then whenever you're ready, you can let your eyes open slowly, but when you do, allow them to open and look ahead with an unfocused gaze for a few moments while your mind relaxes and readjusts.

Breathe naturally and sense the cleansed feeling in your body.

EXERCISE 2: SECOND WARM-UP

Couple by couple, lie down in the center of the room. Take off your shoes. Heads facing out, in the wide part of the circle, feet in the middle, all the feet in the middle touching.

Focus on your breathing and start to let go. Continue to breathe naturally and gently. Put your arms at your sides and let go of the tension in your head. Let your head sink right into the floor, let it go...lose its weight. Lighter and lighter.

Starting with your brow, begin to relax, wrinkle it and unwrinkle it for a minute, so that it's very relaxed. Squeeze your eyes, then let them go. Tighten up your nose, wiggle it around and let it go. Be aware of your cheeks, and relax them...and your mouth, tense it and let go. Tense the muscles of your chin, and your jaw, and then let them go.

And now your shoulders, let them sink right into the floor, first your left one and then your right one and now your back. Tense it, if it helps, before you relax it. Feel the weight of your back go into the floor. Let your waist go into the floor, relax it. And now your stomach, tense those muscles, let them go. And your pelvis, tense the muscles very, very tightly, and then let them go.

Now your thighs, tense them, very tightly, and let go. And now, the lower part of your legs, your calves, tense them, let go. Now your arms, first the upper part of your arms, tense the muscles and relax them. And the lower part of your arms, tense and let them go.

Focus your hands, wiggle your fingers, and let them melt into the floor. And now, lie still, relaxed, let your body sink into the floor and the earth below it...let your mind go...

EXERCISE 3: THE UNFOLDING ROSE

This exercise is adapted from a psychosynthesis technique and will be useful throughout the pregnancy, as well as during labor. The symbol of the flower has been used in both East and West to denote the inner self; the spiritual self. In China, it has been the "Golden Flower"; in India and Tibet, the lotus; in Europe and Persia, the rose. The flower is rooted in the earth, and nourished by the water and the sun. Its development from bud to fully opened bloom parallels the pregnancy process.

Lie down in a comfortable place, or sit in a chair. Close your eyes. Visualize a tightly closed green rosebud. Then move back along the stem until you come to the main branch. Imagine the whole bush with all its leaves and branches and buds, with its roots growing out of the earth.

Then move slowly back to the bud. Imagine the rose opening very slowly, revealing the tip of a delicate pink flower. Watch the flower slowly unfold.

Become the rose. The sun is shining on you. Its warmth hastens your blossoming. Gentle dew covers the surface of your petals and the sun is reflected through the droplets of water. The air caresses you. A gentle breeze ruffles the surface of your petals. The sun fills you with its energy and you open still further. Your sweet, delicate scent is released. You continue to unfold, expanding until you are completely open—in full bloom. Open to all around you.

Remember to speak very slowly when leading an exercise! And leave time in between ideas for the images to develop.

EXERCISE 4: SENSING YOUR ENVIRONMENT

Get comfortable, close your eyes, take a few very deep breaths. As you inhale and exhale, slowly follow your breath through your body and out again. Concentrate your mind on your breath. Be aware of your feelings and sensations but don't judge your thoughts, simply allow them to be there and then let go of those feelings and thoughts.

Sense your stillness and then, as you lift your hand, feel how everything changes. Lie still again and then move your foot. Again sense what happens in your body. Is it only movement? Is there sound? Is there a shift of color or form in your mind's eye? Wiggle your waist. What happens?

Touch your clothing and feel the differences of textures. Do different colors feel different? Touch your skin. How does that feel? Focus on the scent in the room. What does it smell like? Have you been aware of it right along? Does it remind you of anything?

Focus again on your breathing. Be aware of the movement it generates in your body. Be aware of your breath and energy moving out of your body into the room and mingling with the flow of others' energy and becoming part of the sound, smell and movement of the room.

When you are ready, open your eyes slowly and look around the room. Be sensitive to color, form, movement, texture, smell and to the feelings they provoke in you. Continue to use this awareness as you interact with others to understand how these perceptions affect you in the course of your day.

Being aware of your feelings and attitudes on a conscious level can enable you to choose other than simply "react". We mediate our feelings and responses all day long, we're hardly aware we're doing it.

Attuning to your environment—to home, workplace, store, city suburb, country—enables you to have a healthier interaction with it.Even though you find a particular place doesn't suit you, becoming aware of its components and the feelings it arouses allows you to deal with your feelings about it. Often external change is not possible. Internal change is. You'll find yourself relating to your environment quite differently as a result.

EXERCISE 5: GETTING ACQUAINTED

As the group sits in a circle, each person can introduce him or herself briefly, saying whatever each feels important to share. After each person has spoken, you can spend a few minutes learning each other's names. Everyone in turn says their name and turns to the next person, who repeats the preceding names and then says his or her name. For example: "You're John. You're Susan. You're Bill. I'm Leni…" until the last person in the circle has repeated all the names of the people that have preceded her or him. It sounds difficult and maybe embarrassing, but it works well, not only for learning everyone's name, but also for getting people laughing and in a lighter, relaxed state.

EXERCISE 6: GUIDED FANTASY—WATCHING THOUGHTS

Close your eyes and get into a comfortable position…Be aware of the thoughts, words, or images going through your mind.

Imagine that you are in a large room, with two ample doorways on opposite walls. Imagine that your thoughts and images come into this room through one doorway and then go out of the room through the other doorway. Simply watch your thoughts as they move into the room. Let them remain in this room for a while and then move out again. Don't get attached to them. Let them exist apart from you. Simply view them from afar. Observe them…

What are they like? What do they do while they're in the room? How do they come in? How do they go out? Do they rush in and out? Or do they settle into the room gradually so that you can see them separately and clearly?

What happens if you close the exit door? Now open it again…Now close the entrance door and notice what happens…Open it again…Now close both doors and notice what happens…Open them up again…Now close both doors at once and collect a few of your thoughts to bring them back to this room with us…

When you have gathered them, collected them, examine them as carefully as you can…What are they like? How do they act? What do they do now? How do you feel towards these thoughts and how do they respond to you? Talk to them and let them answer you…Now become your thoughts and continue the dialogue…Let all the thoughts bump into each other…Let one emerge...and hold it...Look at it from all sides...When you are ready, open your eyes. And share what's been happening.

EXERCISE 7: MASSAGE CIRCLES

An Opening Exercise for the Beginning of the Evening

The group sits on the floor in a circle, alternating men and women, with new partners on either side. All join hands and close eyes, sitting quietly as they are led through a relaxation exercise. After about five minutes, each person does a half turn to the left and is sitting behind another. Each person massages the head, neck and back of the person in front of them, touching gently yet with depth. Enjoy it yourself—your feelings will communicate. Loving touch invites response. After about seven minutes, everyone reverses and massages the person who has just massaged them. Touching and being touched has many complexities. When, how, how much, what precedes touching, may mean something different to each person. What seems true for all is the message of love and caring.

EXERCISE 8: GROUP ROCK

This exercise expresses affection and caring and also evokes trusting feelings from the person who is being rocked. It's an especially good exercise for men, but nurturing for everyone.

The person to be rocked lies on the floor, and closes her/his eyes. Each member of the group kneels down and puts their hands under a section of the body that they will lift—one person takes the head, another one a shoulder, another the waist, another the hips, another the lower leg, another the feet and so forth, distributing the weight evenly among the group. Then the group lifts the person slowly in a horizontal position as high as they can and rocks them gently back and forth slowly and rhythmically as long as it is comfortable—taking quite a bit of time. When they are ready, they gradually lower the person to the floor, chanting, singing or humming in accompaniment to the movement. The rocked person should lie quietly afterward, absorbing the feelings. This can be done for any group member who requests it, or one member might ask another if she/he would like to be rocked during a stressful evening.

EXERCISE 9: TRUST CIRCLE

One person stands in the center of a circle formed by a group of about six to eight members. The person in the middle closes her/his eyes and relaxing completely, allows her/himself to be passed around the circle from person to person. If the person is heavy, two people may hold the person as they are being passed. She/he may be turned when passed or held for a moment and hugged. The important thing is to relax and allow oneself to be supported by the group.

EXERCISE 10: BLIND WALK

Partners take turns closing their eyes and allowing themselves to be guided wordlessly through the space, trusting that their partners will take care of them. They may lead each other up or downstairs, or sit their partners down, and guide them through different sound, smell and touch experiences—either outside or inside.

This sequence can be followed by a walk with another person also. It is of an entirely different character.

EXERCISE 11: I NEED, I WANT

Sit opposite your partner, each looking directly at the other. Try to maintain eye contact throughout the exercise. If you find you are avoiding holding your partner's gaze, stop for a minute and be aware of the feelings you have when you begin to withdraw.

Each of you take a turn listing all the things you need. Start each sentence with "I need." Your partner will write your list as you state your needs. Get them all out...take about five minutes...When you have exhausted them, start again and exchange "I need" with "I want." Try to consider which are essential to you and which can be eliminated. You may feel that having some emotional needs satisfied seems as important as food and water. That may be so for you...just try to be discriminating about your unique needs. Do the same with "I want."

After you have each had your turn, discuss what you felt about your experience throughout this exercise and about your reaction to your partner's needs and wants. What did you discover? Think about the way you satisfy each other's needs. Think about the social environment between you. Does it work?

EXERCISE 12:

Try the same exercise with the following words: I Have To, I Choose To.

EXERCISE 13:

I Can't, I Won't.

EXERCISE 14: EXPRESSING AMBIVALENCE

This exercise can be done in two different ways. 1. Each person chooses a partner other than her/his own, either a man or a woman. 2. Each partner should write a list following the instructions below:

Take a few minutes to think of all the reasons why you would like to have a baby and then either tell your partner or write your list. If you are working with a partner, the listener should simply receive what is being said, without responding. After the first person is finished, the other takes a turn.

When both have completed their thoughts, think of all the reasons why you *don't* want to have a baby, and listen to each other again.

After completing this part of the exercise, the whole group can share feelings with each other and couples can either break off in pairs afterward for further discussion or continue to share with the group.

There may be some deep and troubling feelings released that require further work. Ambivalence is an important issue to deal with early in the pregnancy.

EXERCISE 15: INSIDE THE WOMB

This is an exercise that gives you a sense of what it may feel like to be inside the womb.

Form groups of four. Stand close together in a circle with arms around each other. Be still for a few minutes with your eyes closed. Become aware of your breathing, of the rise and fall of your chest...Expand your awareness to include those standing beside you and attune to the rhythm of their breathing...

Open your eyes and with a soft unfocused gaze and, without words, take in all the members of the group...the person opposite you...and those beside you...

One by one, in turn, bend from the waist and put your head between the bodies of your group, first at the level of their hearts and then at the level of their abdomens. The other three, with arms still around each other, form an enfolding circle. Gently rock or sway in rhythm with each other. Remain still and focus on creating a synchronized feeling among the group members.

It is helpful to keep your eyes closed throughout the experience. When you are in the center, take as long as you like to have the experience of being held.

EXERCISE 16: MEDITATING WITH THE BABY

This is an exercise designed to focus on the links between mother and father and unborn baby as a threesome. Each partner in a couple sits facing each other, joins hands and closes their eyes as you begin with a relaxation exercise.

Then with eyes still closed, and hands joined, meditate on yourself as a family, on yourself as partners, as a mother or father. Be aware of the life growing inside the womb. Sense your baby. Get in touch with your individual breathing and then feel the movement between you as a couple. Allow your breath to flow from one to the other and then to the baby until you feel you are in rhythm with each other. Visualize the baby's environment inside the womb and imagine what the baby might be experiencing. Consider its sense of you and of the outside world and what you might be communicating to the baby. Think about your feelings as a mother and as a father and stay in touch with yourselves as a threesome. . .

When you are ready, open your eyes. Take a few minutes in silence and then write a conversation with the baby.

This exercise should be done throughout the pregnancy. During the last three months of the pregnancy, the baby is especially prepared to sense its parents in more complex ways. Transmit feelings of love and welcome.

Patting the pregnant abdomen seems a common and universal way of comforting the unborn—not poking at it—not disturbing it—just communicating through touch, caressing it through touch. Mothers seem to do this instinctively. Fathers can, too.

EXERCISE 17: ONE BECOMING TWO BECOMING THREE

Get into a comfortable position. Close your eyes . . .

Think about your week...how has it been? Think about your pregnant body...the baby inside you...your impending motherhood...And fathers, think about your baby inside your partner's womb and about your own body and your impending fatherhood.

Is there anything that's been special about this week? Has anything been particularly meaningful? Was it related to your pregnant state? Any new or unfamiliar feelings? Either in your body or your emotions? How has it been for you as a couple this week? Is there a particular way in which you have thought about each other this week? Any special way you have interacted? Have you had any thoughts or fantasies about the way it will be when you become three instead of two? Even fleeting thoughts should be paid attention to.

Have you had any dreams this week? Take a minute to recall them. Maybe one will even spring to mind that has been forgotten.

With your eyes still closed, each couple join hands and rest your two hands over the womb. Snuggle closer to each other if that feels better...Without sharing it right now with each other, each of you become aware of your baby and have a conversation or communicate in whatever personal way feels right.

With eyes still closed, start to share this experience and the happenings of the week, and the feelings you are now having.

This exercise can be used throughout the pregnancy. Read to your baby in the womb. Sing to it.

EXERCISE 18: AMBIVALENCE

As human beings we have the gift of choice. The choices we make in the present determine our future. Being conscious of choices allows us to create a direction for our lives. The issue of ambivalence revolves around choices. Making them thoughtfully and facing the conflicts that emerge honestly, not only affects one's own life but the lives of others. Choosing to have a child is a serious undertaking, expanding in some ways, limiting in others. Many years of responsibility follow. Nurturing a child, caring for it, educating it takes love, time, money and commitment.

This is an exercise that can be used before conception, early in the pregnancy, and beyond, whenever the issue arises anew.

It is often difficult and perhaps even painful to confront some of the following questions. They are, however, very important to the future of the family you are starting. The clearer you can be with yourselves and the more open with each other, the easier it will be for you in the future.

Sit together as a couple Get into a comfortable position and use one of the relaxation exercises to quiet your mind. With your eyes closed, have one member of the couple read the following questions aloud. Then, with your eyes open and paper and pencil in hand, write down your response to a few questions or to all, if there is time. Think about your answers and let them be the basis of a discussion with the group:

- How do you view your own future? What do you want to achieve in your life?

- How does having a family affect those goals?

- Do you have enough money to have children?

- How do you like the feeling of being pregnant?

- Why do you want a child? What does it mean to you?

- How do you see your life changing? Is it what you want? Are you glad you're pregnant?

- Will a loss of freedom affect your relationship?

- Will having your child hamper your plans for a career, travel, or anything else you want to do?

- Can I depend on my partner in the difficult moments?

- Will our standard of living fall?

- How many children do we want?

- Will we have to move? Can we afford to move?

- Where do we want to live that will suit family life?

- Should we both work? If we don't, will we have enough money?

- Are you grown up enough in your attitudes to be the responsible one?

- Does becoming a mother/father bring good feelings about the future of worrisome ones? Or both?

- How do you feel about the mothering/fathering received?

- As a pregnant woman do you feel helpless and dependent? Do you resent this feeling?

- As a father-to-be do you feel overwhelmed by future responsibilities?

- Can we both get maternity/paternity leave for 6 weeks to 3 months when the baby is born?

- What about the new triangle? Have I had experience of other triangle?

- Are you glad or sorry you're having a baby now? Is it a convenient time? Was this pregnancy planned?

- Can you still handle your job and be a good mother or father?

- Are you realistic about what it's going to be like to have a child?

EXERCISE 19: BIRTH MEDITATION AND DRAWING EXERCISE

Lie on the floor next to your partner and form a group wheel—a mandala, with the hands touching in the center of the wheel.

Close your eyes. Fathers, place your hands over the womb, over the baby. Mothers, place your hand on your partner's hand...Become aware of your breathing. Gently, breathe in and out, slowly...in and out...breathe in rhythm with each other and be aware of the baby's rhythms. Inhale...exhale...deep breaths. Fill your lungs and let the breath empty completely.

Visualize a ball of energy—a ball of light—in the middle of your forehead and hold it there...Now start that ball of energy moving clockwise in a spiral around inside your head, moving downward, circling your throat and around inside your shoulders, then around into your heart...Then let it circle around your heart again and around the arm that is placed on the womb...The energy ball spiraling around your arm...into your hand...the hand that is connected to each other and to the baby. Let it come to rest there...the two balls of energy merging...Remain quiet as long as it feels comfortable, perhaps three minutes.

Now gather your own energy ball again and spiral it back through and up around your heart, slowly circling your shoulders...your throat and back of the middle of your forehead...Let it fade slowly away.

When you are ready, open your eyes and get comfortable. Sit up. Take one piece of paper and share a box of crayons and draw together as a couple anything you want but be sure to include your baby in the picture. Use color, shape and images to express the feelings evoked. After you are finished, share with each other: How did it feel? Was it cooperative? How much space did each take up? How do you like your drawing? Then share, if you like, with the whole group. Do this exercise often during the pregnancy and see how your attitudes change.

EXERCISE 20: NAMELESS CHILD

Lie down. Close your eyes. After a relaxation exercise, listen to these words and move with them.

There is a mountain of gold. When the sun's rays strike it, it is irritating to look at. It is surrounded by red, green, orange, purple and pink clouds, wafted gently by the wind. Around the mountain fly thousands of copper-winged birds with silver heads and iron beaks. A ruby sun rises in the east and a crystal moon sets in the west. The whole earth is covered with pearl-dust snow. Suddenly, a luminous child without a name comes into being.

> The golden mountain is dignified,
> The sunlight is blazing red,
> Dreamlike clouds of many colors float across the sky.
> In the place where metal birds croak,
> The instantaneously born child can find no name.

Because the child has no father, the child has no family line. The child has never tasted milk because the child has no mother. There is no one to play with because the child has neither brother nor sister. Having no house to live in, the child has no crib. Since the child has no nanny, the child has never cried. There is no civilization, so the child has no toys. Since there is no point of reference, the child has never found a self. The child has never heard spoken language, so the child has never experienced fear.

The child walks in every direction, but does not come across anything. The child sits down slowly on the ground. Nothing happens. The colorful world seems sometimes to exist and sometimes not. The child gathers a handful of pearl-dust and slowly lets it trickle through his fingers. The child gathers another handful and slowly takes it into his mouth. Hearing the pearl dust crunch between its teeth, the child gazes at the ruby sun setting and the crystal moon rising. Suddenly, there's a whole galaxy of stars and the child lies on its back to admire their patterns. The child falls into a deep sleep, but has no dreams.

> The child's world has no beginning or end.
> To him, colors are neither beautiful nor ugly.
> He has no preconceived notion of birth and death.
>
> The golden mountain is solid and unchanging,
> The ruby sun is all-pervading,
> The crystal moon watches over millions of stars,
> The child exists without preconceptions.
>
> *Dharmas Without Blame*, Chogyam Trungpa,

Become the baby curled and floating in the womb. Surround yourself with these sounds, as if nothing else exists.

Afterward discuss your experience as a group.

EXERCISE 21: GUIDED FANTASY OF PREGNANCY AND BIRTH

I have used this exercise with groups as large as one hundred, or more, with wonderful results. Be sure to lead it slowly and with many quiet spaces for people to interact.

The group will form families of three and each one will decide which role they would like to play. There should be a mother, father and a baby (a fetus) in this experience of pregnancy and birth. You can choose to play whatever part you wish and do some role reversing so that men can have the sense of being mothers, women of being fathers and those who choose to be babies can be whatever gender they wish. If there are more people than a three-person family accommodates, expand it into foursomes and have twins in some families.

When you have chosen your families, find a roomy place on the floor where your family can stretch out and lie down close to each other, holding hands or being in contact with each other in a way that feels comfortable. If you like you can have music in the background; Dr. Hajime Murooka's "Lullaby From The Womb" (Mother's Heartbeat—and Sounds from the Body Arteries), or Michael Jean Jarre's "Oxygen" are good ones.

Get comfortable...relax as fully as you can, using one of the earlier relaxation exercises.

Mothers, enfold the babies in a position that will be comfortable for a period of time. Find a position that allows the baby to feel in close body contact to you, enclosed and symbiotic. Fathers, stay close, although you may be more active in your positions and will probably move around more. Find a position that is in relationship to the mother and baby. And babies, curl up comfortably with your mother so you feel enfolded...in the womb of the mother.

Now the baby begins to focus on this experience and parents also will focus on this experience, trying to create it as an ideal experience for all of you—to design your own emotional birth environment—you the baby and you the mother and father, collectively creating a positive birth environment inside and outside the womb right here.

Imagine that conception has taken place—that the fertilized egg has begun to divide, splitting first into two cells, then into four. After a week, it has become a ball of cells. The baby is growing rapidly. Mothers don't yet know that they are pregnant.

Babies, sense yourselves as tiny fetuses attached to the wall of the womb, growing and expanding. And talk to your parents for a few moments about what is happening for you as you are becoming...Focus on the environment in which you are living and on your parents beyond that environment. Sense the feelings that you are being imbued with and that you want to carry along—the qualities that you are sensing from your mother and father. Tell them out loud now about your sense of yourself coming to life as a combination of these two parents. Tell them about the weaknesses and strengths that are forming you, the feminine side, the masculine side—all that you sense. With your eyes still closed, tell them what you are feeling.

Parents, don't answer your baby or get involved in conversation just now, simply listen. Let the baby experience the wonder of its beginning. When the baby is finished talking, parents can talk to each other about the pregnancy. Mothers, you have just learned that you are pregnant. Start to talk about what that means to you. Fathers, begin to respond about the way you feel and what it means to you, about your excitement, your fears, your needs, and, perhaps, even your ambivalence. Whatever you are experiencing. Babies, just listen without being involved in your parents' conversation.

Babies, you are now three months old. Inside the womb, you are learning what it is like to live in between these two people. You are beginning to sense when your needs aren't being fully met and when they are. Babies, tell your parents what will make you feel totally secure and loved by your parents. And then, parents, try to accommodate the needs that your baby has expressed t you—each in your own way.

Babies, you are now six months old. Mothers, you have felt the flutterings of life for more than a month. The baby is a reality. Parents, what are you feeling? Are you able to ask for what you need? Do you know what you need from each other or others. What aren't you getting? Tell each other now what is happening for you.

Babies, simply listen to your parents' conversation without interacting with them and sense the mood and the quality of their relationship. You are quite active now. You have found your fingers and are even sucking them; you sip the fluids in the womb; you hear sounds in your mother's body and from outside her body, many vibrations...After your parents are finished talking to each other, tell them what you are experiencing in the womb, what your environment is like and how their relationship affects you. Also what you would like...to be held more closely, perhaps to have more relaxed time together? Whatever.

Parents, be very sensitive and aware of your baby's needs as you sense them, and of your own needs, too. Tell the baby how you feel about its presence. What your hopes and expectations are. And your fears.

Fathers, how are you feeling? Isolated or involved? Will you share with the mother and the baby? Try to work out something that feels better.

We are now about eight months into pregnancy. The birth is drawing near. The baby is getting quite heavy now. It's a little harder to reach mother, physically. Her shape has changed a lot. Would you share some of the problems about that with each other and the baby? Mother, are you feeling very sexy? Would you share your thoughts and feelings about that? Father, are you feeling turned on by mother at this stage? What's interfering for you? Talk about it together.

Babies, how are you feeling about your environment? Is it getting crowded? Are you impatient? Do you move around a lot—or respond to the life around you? How? Tell your parents your feelings.

As a unit, as a family, try to meet everyone's individual needs. See if that is possible as you are near the ninth month—the end of the pregnancy. Mother, how are you doing with all your needs? What are they? Can father help you in any way? Could you speak to the baby about it? What are your feelings now as you are about to separate from your baby? In the next few minutes, tell each other what is happening for each of you.

Tomorrow is the day the baby will be born. Parents, talk to each other about what your needs are for the birth. Baby, begin to fantasize the environment in which you would like to be born. I want you to begin to construct in your mind what you each need—in terms of environment—people and physical space, in terms of the colors or light or darkness, in terms of sound and textures and temperature. Babies, decide what would make you feel welcome in the world. Let it take shape in your mind. Parents, tell each other what you need and envision and then baby, share with them what you need to make you feel nurtured and welcomed.

The three of you together share out loud what the ideal environment should be and what you want.

Are you feeling anxious or expectant or strong? What are you feeling?

It is beginning—the mother and baby know it is time for the baby to be born. The baby begins its movement through the birth canal and each of you plays your part in a way that allows this birth to be joyful. Stay in touch with each other as the birth occurs. Continue to tell each other what you need—the baby, mother, father—as the birth progresses.

Welcome the baby when it is born. Snuggle it, cuddle it, caress it.

Babies, continue to share what you need from your parents and the environment, what you sense you need to have around you. Will the mother share what she needs, after this ordeal or this joyous experience? Will the father remain in contact and assess his needs...what he senses he can give or not give...what he senses is needed from him?

Slowly begin to resettle yourselves comfortable as a family and talk to each other about this experience. Stay together, in close contact with each other as you talk a few minutes.

Then share as a large group and tell how it went.

EXERCISE 22: DRAWING THE BODY

Each person lies down on a life-sized piece of paper (a roll of wrapping paper is good) while another traces around her/his body shape. Each person then takes her/his paper image and fills in the inside space with a colored version of feelings, organs, bones, circulatory systems, emotions, whatever they feel is inside. After everyone is finished, after about twenty to thirty minutes, each person explains her/his picture to the others and gets feedback from the group. It may surprise you to hear yourself describe what is inside your body.

EXERCISE 23: WHO AM I?

Each of us embodies so many different aspects that it is helpful to set down all of the roles and qualities that are part of our lives. It will give you an enriched sense of how you view yourself and how you order those roles and qualities. You can see how the labels of others affect your sense of your own unique perceptions of yourself. You can also sense the ways those role boundaries may inhibit growth and development of a fuller self.

Choose a partner and, in turn, each of you list aloud the answers to the question, "Who Am I?" while your partner writes down your list. When you have exhausted all the "I am's" you can possibly think of, have your partner read them aloud. Then do the same for your partner. After both of you have completed your lists, take a few minutes to discuss what you have felt about the list you each generated. They will probably start with "I am a woman," "I am an American," "I am a daughter," and move into more unique aspects.

Follow this part of the exercise with a list of the qualities you feel you have, both the ones you're pleased with and perhaps some that get in your way: "I am generous," "I am shy," "I am self-disciplined"...

You might go on to some more imaginative ways in which you envision yourself: "I am a fast-moving river," "I am a majestic mountain," "I am a knife that cuts clean," "I am an elf."

EXERCISE 24: I AM A HOUSE (PERSONAL SPACE)

Imagine you are a house. Describe the house. Walk around the outside of the house. Observe its color and shape. Is it opened or closed? Describe the walls and windows. Of what material are they made? What is its setting? Is it isolated or set among other houses or…How does it look?

How many entrances does it have? Notice the shapes of the doors. Describe them. Open the door, walk in, walk through the space and observe it in detail. Then describe it. Is it full or empty? What is its decoration? Does it have an attic or cellar? Does one or the other evoke feelings? Move through all its spaces. Touch it, smell it, sense the ambience. Are there people other than yourself in it? Are there changes you would like to make? People you would like to bring in? What are the colors? What are the shapes? Which rooms are favorites? Why? Which do you live in?

The state of my house seems to reflect the state of my mind and my emotions right now.

This exercise will probably evoke different images each time you do it. That is one of its advantages. It is also one you can do alone, as well as with others. Relax, get comfortable. Listen to a recording of the exercise, record or write your response.

EXERCISE 25: FAMILY RECOLLECTIONS

- What did your parents, grandparents, aunts, uncles, sisters, brothers, cousins, tell you about your birth? What did you feel about what you were told?

- What story did your parents tell you about how you were named? What did you feel about this?

Be your parents describing these things to you, through role playing. Were there any "don't be you" injunctions, like: "You almost killed me when I had you," "I suffered a lot,"...

EXERCISE 26: NAMING

Were you named after someone? If so, were you expected to replace someone or adopt their personalities? Is your name masculine or feminine? Was your namesake of the opposite sex? What qualities do you associate with your name?—first, middle, surname. What qualities did they associate with your name? Have you adopted those qualities? Do you like your name? Have you always?

EXERCISE 27: CHILDHOOD ATTITUDES

Start with a relaxation exercise as you lie in a circle with your heads meeting in the middle and your feet pointed to the edge of the circle you have formed.

Then, with your eyes still closed, move back through time and sense yourself as a young child—at six, seven, eight or so. Recall your mother and father and your family setting. What did you know about pregnancy and birth? Did you have a younger sibling? What was said to you specifically about birth, about where babies came from? Did someone else talk about birth to you? What filters through? Take as much time as you need to reexperience those feelings and then when you are ready, open your eyes and while you are still lying in the circle, begin to share your recollections.

EXERCISE 28: INTERVIEWING YOUR MOTHER AND FATHER

During pregnancy, it can be very useful to spend some time talking to your mother and father about their recollections of pregnancy, labor and your birth. Although it is usually not a sub-

pregnancy, labor and your birth. Although it is usually not a subject that we discuss with our parents, since it is often a taboo subject in some families about which we couldn't ask or discuss, nevertheless, you will probably be surprised, as will she and he, by how fresh the memory is. Very often birth patterns are repeated from generation to generation, so it would be important to be aware of what preceded your experience so that you might avoid some unconscious programming.

You might propose the idea to your mother and father ahead of time so that they can begin to think about it and memories can be stirred. Some women may be reluctant to recall difficult, lonely or painful times, so be sensitive to what your mother is feeling. She may need reassurance form you about why you are asking after all these years, so broach the subject with care. She'll probably be delighted to re-remember for her own sake, as will your father. Siblings can be a source also. they may also be helpful in recalling family attitudes and happenings. Their memories may be quite different form yours.

Maybe it will be a monologue or perhaps a dialogue. It might be good to have a few definite things that you want to know in case you adapt an interview style. The group might discuss together what you would like to ask.

You might want to ask:

- What her pregnancy was like

- What kind of medical care she received when pregnant

- Whether she had any preparation for labor

- What your father's attitude was

- What her recollection was of the environment of birth

- What her labor was like and who was with her

- Her memory of the birth

- What happened right after and in the weeks that followed

- Were you nursed? Why yes or no.

You might tape the conversation or write down what happens. It's very helpful to do so. It's surprising how much goes by when you don't record things. And it's often informative to listen to changes of tone of voice and abrupt shifts in conversation after you absorb the content. They all have their own meaning.

One way you might bring the interviews back into the group would be to simply have the whole group report their stories back one evening and share about what you learned. Another way would be to meet in two groups for part of the evening. One for the men and one for the women. It is often a good way to heighten intimacy beyond the couple. Different things may be brought out in this way.

Both groups may be able to discuss sensitive issues they find difficult to mention in the full group. Often questions of sexuality are more easily explored at the beginning in an all-men or all-women group and certainly the sexuality of pregnancy is a ripe area to be explored. This might be a good opportunity to begin discussions that can later be shared in the full group.

Follow a similar procedure with your father or other members of your family.

EXERCISE 29: KEEPING A JOURNAL

Discussion about keeping a journal. What might it include?

- Feelings on awakening and at the end of the day

- Dreams, fantasies, body sensations

- Feelings, thoughts at different points of the day

- Feelings about the changes in your life now and in the future

- Recording important happenings in the day

- Drawing, writing poetry, and/or stream of consciousness writing.

Beginning the journal:

- Write a brief entry for last week

- Write a brief entry for today

- Those who would like to can read their entries to the group

EXERCISE 30: CROSSROADS IN THE JOURNAL— STEPPING-STONES

This is an exercise I learned from Ira Progroff's *At a Journal Workshop,* one of the methods I explored in the course of my own journey. It is an exercise that can be done often. (Following the direction of this book can be a rich and fruitful method in itself for those to whom journals appeal.)

With paper and pencil in hand, take a few minutes to relax. Become still. Focus on your breathing. Empty your mind. When you feel quiet, begin to reflect on important events in your life that led to this moment. You can reach back as far as you like. To your birth, if that feels right. Simply allow images of people, places, events, feelings to arise without judging them. When you come to a crossroad—a stepping-stone—when you recall making a choice between two directions, reflect upon it, and another and another. You will be drawing out particular strands of your unique tapestry. Move back through time—your life— and select ten or twelve threads that connect you to this pregnant moment.

After ten or fifteen minutes of writing, the group can share their stories.

EXERCISE 31: A GAME OF WORD ASSOCIATION

Write out as many similes as you can dream up for each of the following words and then add some words of your own:

Birth, a mother, a father, a baby, an environment for birth, breasts, blood, a doctor, a nurse...Example: Birth is like the heavens shaking.

Create as many spontaneous images as you can—funny ones, whimsical, logical and illogical ones.

When you have a list of about eight to ten for each, read them aloud couple by couple. It's intriguing to see the overlaps and the differences and the connections you yourself have made.

Another version of this exercise can be to simply free-associate to these words, writing down your quick responses: blood, sex, breasts, pain, pregnancy...

EXERCISE 32: BECOMING YOUR MOTHER AND FATHER

Close your eyes and go back to your youth. Choose an age that was important to you, around ten, eleven, or twelve. Visualize your mother. What does she look like? What is she wearing? How does she walk? What is the tone of her voice? When you feel you have a strong sense of her, open your eyes and stand up. Begin to circulate around the room taking on the role of your mother. Become her. Walk the way you remember her walking, talk the way she talked. Act her part as well as you can. Move among the other "mothers" and talk to each other about pregnancy and birth. You can imagine that each of you is pregnant or that you have just given birth. You will find that it is quite easy to take on her physical and emotional characteristics.

After about five to ten minutes, switch and become your father. Take time to close your eyes again and get into visualizing him as you did your mother before you begin to act the role.

EXERCISE 33: ARCHETYPAL MOTHERS AND FATHERS

Focus on the archetypal mother. Think about all the good mothers you have known and the qualities they embodied.

Focus on the archetypal father. Thank about all the good fathers you have known and the qualities they embodied.

EXERCISE 34: FATHER'S FANTASY OF BEING PREGNANT

The men in the group sit in a circle in the center of the room and imagine that *they* are the pregnant mothers. Stuffing a small pillow under their shirts can help the role reversal.

Close your eyes. Breathe gently and naturally, allowing your breath to rise and fall without needing to change it. Feel your belly with your hands. Feel the roundness of it, the firmness of it. Feel the pressure of the womb against your chest and the bulge resting on your lap. Your belly has been growing gradually for the past months—you are seven months pregnant. You are feeling full and ripe. The baby is moving around inside you, kicking, turning, making its presence felt. Share with the other "mothers" in the circle what you are feeling.

EXERCISE 35: COUPLE MEDITATION—GETTING YOUR NEEDS MET

Close your eyes. Get comfortable. Sit opposite each other. Empty your mind of thoughts as best you can. Focus your attention on your breathing as your chest moves in and out, and as your abdomen rises and falls, feel your breathing deepen. When you feel still, join hands with your spouse, hold each other gently and, with eyes still closed, focus your attention on each other....Is there something you would like to ask for—more attention? More privacy? Less of something?

When you are ready, open your eyes and continue to look at each other without exchanging words. When you have had enough quiet time, share with each other verbally what you would like from the other…Each of you take five minutes or so, without interruption from your partner.

When you are finished with this part of the exercise, share with each other the feelings and thoughts that were occurring as the other one spoke. Stay in touch with your body reactions throughout, making note of how you feel and where you feel it. Share with the whole group when you are finished exchanging with each other, if you care to.

EXERCISE 36: GIVING AND TAKING

The group sits on the floor in a circle. One person who has trouble receiving sits in the center of the circle and sits with their eyes closed. Each person gives to them, in turn, nonverbally, without words. The person in the center of the circle has their eyes closed. Another may take their place. Afterward, everyone shares their feelings. Often, after a couple has ventilated angry feelings towards each other, we form a "love" circle with the couple standing in the middle and the others surrounding them closely in a group hug.

EXERCISE 37: I APPRECIATE, I RESENT

"I Appreciate" is a lovely and important follow-up for "I Resent" and might be combined as an exercise.

Each member of a couple sits opposite each other and, one at a time, taking about five minutes each, tells the other what they resent about the other's behavior.

"I appreciate" follows the same procedure, and partners tell each other in turn what they appreciate about the other.

EXERCISE 38: A FANTASY SHOPPING TRIP—GIVING AND TAKING

Close your eyes and get comfortable…Imagine you are wandering down a street, looking in the shop windows, trying to find a wonderful gift for your partner. Choose a place anywhere in the world...be free and fanciful about your choices. Imagine the time of day...and the weather...and continue walking in the scene you are creating.

Visualize your partner, think about what he or she likes, what would please him or her...When you find the place that carries the sort of gift you might like to choose, open the door, if there is a door. Walk inside, look around and choose a gift that is very particular for your partner. It may be an object, a think, or it may be a quality that embodies your feeling. The gift will express some of the feelings that you have about him or her. Choose one gift of maybe two. Perhaps you will have to go to another shop for the second gift. When you have your gift, open your eyes. As a group, go around the circle and give your partner your imaginary gift and tell him or her what it means to you.

Other suggestions for couples on their own at home throughout the pregnancy:

- Draw your baby once a month, or even more often,. either individually or together. Observe your feelings as your baby grows in the bomb. Use the drawings as a window to your changing attitudes and feelings.

- Invite the baby's grandparents to record family histories and favorite family stories for the baby.

- Prospective fathers and mothers can read to their babies in the womb. Fathers can make a tape of a favorite children's story so that it can be played when they aren't there. It is especially fruitful during the last six or seven weeks of pregnancy. Babies seem to remember and connect.

An experimental study was conducted by Gina Kolala about learning in the womb. Twice a day during the last month and a half of pregnancy, sixteen women read aloud Dr. Seuss' *The Cat in the Hat* to their babies in the womb. After birth, tapes of their mother's voices were played for the babies. *The Cat in the Hat* and another story, not read to them during pregnancy, *The King, the Mice and the Cheese* were heard by the newborns. There was a preference for *The Cat in the Hat* by all babies, indicated by sucking patterns. Researchers conclude that during womb existence babies listen to adult speech and can differentiate and remember the sounds of words.

EXERCISE 39: ASKING—RECEIVING

One father in the group who had an easy time giving and a difficult time receiving was asked to go around the room and ask each person for something that was characteristic of him or her.

Example: 'George, would you give me something? I'd like some of your strength. Barbara, would you give me some of your creativity? Another was asked to share his spontaneity, another protection. If you gave me some of your warmth and protection, I could get rid of this cold shield. To his wife, he said: Would you give me some of your anger, some negativity? It's the one thing you withhold from me.

EXERCISE 40: EXPRESSING FEELINGS

Break up into groups of threes, choosing the people in the group you know least well. One person will be the monologuer, one the listener, one the recorder. Each member of the threesome will have a turn in each role.

The monologuer begins by telling the listener about his/her initial reactions to the pregnancy and about the way those feelings have been evolving. The listener simply listens without response—either in words, or facial or body response. The listener is present as a nonjudgmental mirror. The recorder makes notes of what is being said so that the speaker has another point of observation to refer to. After about five or ten minutes, the roles are switched until each person has had a chance to be the speaker.

When it has moved around the circle, the threesome can share their reactions and observations with their threesome and later with the group as a whole. Do this many times during the months of the group. Everyone will get better at expressing their feelings.

EXERCISE 41: NONVERBAL HAND CONVERSATION

Stand in a circle; hold hands. Stay with your own feelings, yet in touch with each other. Sense each other. Break from the circle and join hands with your spouse. Be with each other nonverbally. Communicate your feelings through your hands. With one hand, shake hands, say hello...play...Then let the hands fight...then let the hands make up...be impatient or teasing— and become loving again...Then say good-bye. Share the feelings that were evoked with the group. They can be quite explosive or amusing or...

EXERCISE 42: TWO MASSAGE EXERCISES

Massage—Sensing, Exploring, Giving and Taking

Intimacy is central to the experience of pregnancy and birth for both partners. Becoming attuned to each other's needs and feelings and bodies through sensing and touching builds a foundation for family times ahead. In the first years, each parent will need to understand the needs of their new baby and be able to express feelings without relying on words.

Giving and receiving through sensitive touching are personal art forms that can enrich every relationship we have. How wonderful it feels to be touched! How much we can understand about another simply through touch. Barriers can be broken through, deep feelings can be expressed, nurturing can occur quite simply.

There are many ways to expand your sensitivity, and some of the books mentioned in the Bibliography will be quite helpful. Here is one exercise from *Your Second Life,* by Gay Gaer Luce, for the group to use in early sessions when they are just getting to know each other. Working with someone less familiar to you can expand your sensitivity to your partner. Move slowly into physical contact, aware of each group member's vulnerable feelings and differences. Share with each other and the group what you each felt.

Back to Back and Face to Face

Settle on the floor with a partner, either your own or another member of the group. The first time you do the exercise it might be best to do it with the person you know least in the group. When you are sitting comfortably with your back against your partner's back, close your eyes and take a few deep breaths. Begin to feel the rhythm of your partner's breathing. As you get into synchrony with your partner's breathing rhythm, sense what he or she may be feeling. Give yourselves a few minutes to be together in this way.

Next, in turn and without speaking to each other, each of you will become the support for the other. One of you lean back against your partner until your head is resting on your partner's head. Relax your body, especially your shoulders. Just allow your partner to support your weight. As you relax and lean back, your partner will slowly begin to straighten his-her back to be a better supporter.

Now begin to roll your back against your partner's and each of you can massage the back of the other as you move against each other's backs, shoulders, neck and head.

After you have switched so that each partner has had a chance to be both supporter and supported, turn around and face each other. Again in turn, wordlessly and with eyes closed, touch each other's faces and gently explore and massage the forehead, around the eyes, the cheeks, the nose and so forth until all of the face has been explored. Take time and sense what your partner may be feeling and what you are feeling yourself as your hands move over your partner's face.

After each of you has had your turn, open your eyes and share your experience with each other and with the group later if you like.

Massage

One person lies on the floor. All the members of the group gather around the person and massage her or him. You can give them a face, back and shoulder, foot or entire body massage. Be gentle, caressing, and nurturing, stroking tenderly yet working into tense muscles.

Another way can be for couples to work on each other in turn. It is a very nurturing way to be with each other.

There are some very good books available on massage technique, several of which are listed in the Bibliography.

EXERCISE 43: CHANTING A NAME

An exercise for a mother or father who needs loving attention.

Sit in the center of a circle formed by the group and, after looking around at each person in the group that is surrounding you, close your eyes and relax. Focus attention on your breathing rhythm first and, then as you become calm, imagine that you are opening the entire surface of your body to receive the vibration of your name...The group starts to chant your name quietly, allowing the sound to develop as it will. Allow it to continue as long as the group feeling is there and until it ends in a natural way.

The sensory experience of having your name chanted is surprising.

EXERCISE 44: LOVE BOMBARDMENT

Several times in the group, after one or another tearfully expressed fear, frustration or distress, we did an exercise called "Love Bombardment," a rather simple, obvious and effective group gesture of affection. All the members of the group surround the person, hold her or him in their arms, cradling, rocking, crooning and relaxing. As you can imagine, it is effective and beautiful and the child in each of us needs this sort of loving attention at times.

EXERCISE 45: VISIT TO THE DOCTOR—A ROLE-PLAYING EXERCISE

Several members of the group act out a typical visit to the doctor. The mother can watch while someone plays her part. Her partner might choose to do that, or someone else. Someone plays the doctor, someone else the nurse or whatever parts the woman who is directing the activity designates. It should follow the details of her actual experience. After she describes her usual visit, she can replay it, this time asking all the questions she forgot to ask, saying all the things she meant to say or was afraid to say. It can be rehearsed several times until she feels clear about her needs. Repetition usually reveals hidden agendas and also increases self-confidence. Fathers can participate in the same way.

EXERCISE 46: REHEARSAL FOR BIRTH

Start with a relaxation exercise. Then with eyes closed, focus on the word *birth*. Allow whatever images, words or feelings to arise...It is the time for the baby to be born...Imagine how the birth might take place. How would you like it to be—for you and for your baby? Visualize the physical place, the people who will be there, the ambience...Where are you? Who is with you? What are they doing? Let the drama unfold. You are the producer-director. It may be a symbol, a whole scenario, a fleeting image. Accept what comes. It will develop in your unconscious and continue to emerge perhaps later in a dream or a waking fantasy—trust your unconscious to work it through.

When you feel satisfied with what is happening in your fantasy, come slowly back to this room and this moment...Tell your partner what you envisioned and then share with the group.

This exercise can be practiced several times before the birth.

EXERCISE 47: WELCOMING THE BABY

The baby is at the center of this transformation that is taking place. This exercise can be used over and over with different feelings evoked each time, I'm sure.

Lie down. Close your eyes and relax in whatever way feels good for you. Take time to unwind and let go. Don't rush into the second part of the exercise until you feel that each part of your body has let go of its tension. Check through your whole body slowly. Are you now relaxed?

Begin to smile, still with your eyes closed. Sense what happens to your mouth as you smile, as your lips elongate, as your cheek muscles tighten to create a smile. Sense all the small changes that occur in your face as your smile gets larger.

How do you feel as you smile? What happens to the rest of your face? And your shoulders and your spine? Move through your body and invite it to participate in the smile. How does that happen for you?

Now, when you feel that your whole being is smiling, envision the baby. Mothers, put your hands over the womb. Fathers, become part of the triangle in whatever way feels comfortable.

When you feel that your heart is in psychic touch with your baby and that your breathing rhythms are coordinated, communicate your pleasure to the baby and tell it what you are feeling about its arrival. Try to transfer all the good feelings that accompany your smiling person to the baby. Tell it how much you love it and how welcome it is and will be.

BIBLIOGRAPHY:
SUGGESTED READING AND RESEARCH
SOURCES

General

Bowlby, John. *Attachment and Loss.* Volume I: *Attachment,* 1969, Volume II: *Separation, Anxiety and Anger,* 1973. New York: Basic Books, 1973.

Campbell, Joseph. *The Power of the Myth.* New York: Anchor Books, 1990.

Condon, William. *Studies of Movements of Babies and Mothers.* The Journal of Nervous and Mental Diseases. Volume 134, pp. 338-347, 1966.

Fodor, Nandor. *The Search for the Beloved.* New York: Hermitage, 1949.

Fromm, Erich. *The Art of Loving.* New York: Harper & Row, 1974.

Grof, Stanislav. *Realms of the Human Unconscious.* New York: Dutton, 1976.

____. *Beyond the Brain: Birth, Death and Transcendence in Psychotherapy.* Albany, NY: State University of New York Press, 1985.

____. *The Adventure of Self-Discovery.* Albany, NY: State University of New York Press, 1988.

Harding, M. Esther. *Women's Mysteries.* New York: Putnam, C.J. Jung Foundation Series, 1971.

Laing, R.D. *The Politics of the Family.* New York: Pantheon, 1971.

____. *The Facts of Life.* New York: Pantheon, 1976.

Janov, Arthur. *The Bond of Power.* New York: Dutton, 1981.

____. *Imprints: The Lifelong Effects of the Birth Experience.* New York: Coward-McCann, 1983.

Leboyer, Frederick. *Birth Without Violence.* New York: Knopf, 1975.

____. *Loving Hands.* New York: Knopf, 1976.

Maslow, Abraham H. *Toward a Psychology of Being.* New York: Van Nostrand Reinhold, 1968.

May, Rollo. *Love and Will.* New York: Norton Inc., 1969.

Mead, Margaret. *Male and Female.* New York: Wm. Morrow, 1975.

Meltzer, David. *Birth.* New York: Ballantine, 1973.

Montagu, Ashley. *Touching: The Human Significance of Skin.* New York: Wiley, 1964.

Newman, E. *The Great Mother.* New York: Pantheon, 1955.

Nilsson, Lennart. *Behold Man.* Boston: Little, Brown, 1973.

Olivier, Marc. *The Psychology of the House.* New York: Thames and Hudson, 1977.

Rank, Otto. *The Trauma of Birth.* New York: Harper/Torchbooks, 1973.

Suzuki, Shunryu. *Zen Mind, Beginner's Mind.* New York: John Weatherhill, 1970.

Weisman, Harry and Kerr, George R. *Fetal Growth and Development.* "Parental Determinants of Postnatal Behavior." New York: McGraw Hill, 1970.

Prenatal/Postnatal Sources

Bibring, Grete, et al. "A Study of the Psychological Processes in Pregnancy and the Earliest Mother-Child Relationship." *Psychoanalytical Studies of the Child,* XVI, 1961.

Bittman, Sam, and Sue Zalk. *Expectant Fathers.* New York: Hawthorn Books, 1978.

Brazelton, T. Berry. *On Becoming a Family: The Growth of the Attachments.* New York: Delacorte, 1981.

____. *What Every Baby Knows.* Reading, MA: Addison-Wesley, 1987.

Caplan, Gerald. *Concepts of Mental Health and Consultation,* p. 6, No. 373, U.S. Government Printing Office, 1959.

Colman, Arthur D., and Libby L. Colman. *Pregnancy: The Psychological Experience.* New York: Seabury Press, 1971.

Deutsch, Helene. *The Psychology of Women. Volume II.* New York: Research Books, 1947.

Heinowitz, Jack. *Pregnant Fathers.* New York: A Spectrum Book, 1982.

Newton, Niles. *Maternal Emotions.* New York: Paul B. Hoeber, Inc., 1963.

Shapiro, Jerrold Lee. *When Men Are Pregnant.* San Luis Obispo: Impact, 1987.

Sidoli, Mara. *The Unfolding Self.* Boston: Sigo Press, 1990.

Stern, Daniel. *The Interpersonal World of the Infant, A View From Psychoanalysis and Developmental Psychology. New York:* Basic Books, 1985.

____. *Diary of a Baby.* New York: Basic Books, 1990.

Wickes, Frances G. *Inner World of Childhood.* Boston: Sigo Press, 1990.

____. *Inner World of Choice.* Boston: Sigo Press, 1990.

Aspects of Pregnancy and Birth

American College of Obstetricians and Gynecologists. *Family-Centered Maternity/Newborn Care in Hospitals.* One E. Wacker Drive, Suite 270, Chicago, Illinois 60601.

Arms, Suzanne. *Immaculate Deception.* Boston: Houghton Mifflin, 1975.

Bean, Constance. *Methods of Childbirth*. Garden City, NY: Doubleday, 1972.

Boston Women's Health Book Collective. *Ourselves and Our Children*. New York: Random House, 1978.

Bradley, Robert A. *Husband-Coached Childbirth*. New York: Harper & Row, 1974.

Chamberlain, David. *Babies Remember Birth*. Los Angeles: Jeremy P. Tarcher, 1988.

Coleman, Arthur and Libby Coleman. *Pregnancy: The Psychological Experience*. New York: Seabury Press, 1973.

Day, Beth and Margaret Liby. *The Secret World of the Baby*. New York: Random House, 1968.

Dick-Read, Grantly. *Childbirth Without Fear*. New York: Harper & Row, 1984.

Feher, Leslie. *The Psychology of Birth: Foundations of Human Personality*. London: Souvenir Press, 1980.

Flanagan, Geraldine. *The First Nine Months of Live*. New York: Simon & Schuster, 1962.

Hendricks, Gay and Hendricks, Kathlyn. "Techniques for Dealing With Prenatal and Perinatal Issues in Therapy: A Bodymind Approach." *Pre- and Perinatal Psychology Journal* 1 (3), pp. 230-238.

Hotchner, Tracy. *Pregnancy and Childbirth*. New York: Avon, 1979.

Howells, John, ed. *Modern Perspectives in Psycho-obstetrics*. New York: Brunner-Mazel, 1972.

Kelley-Buchanan, Christine. *Peace of Mind During Pregnancy. An A-Z Guide to the Substances That Could Affect Your Unborn Baby*. New York: Facts on File Publications, 1989.

Kitzinger, Sheila. *The Experience of Childbirth*. London: Penguin Books, 1987.

____. *Being Born:* New York: Grossett & Dunlap, 1986.

____. *Your Baby, Your Way: Making Pregnancy Decisions and Birth Plans*. New York: Pantheon, 1987.

Klaus, Marshall and John Kennell. *Maternal-Infant Bonding*. St. Louis, MO: C.V. Mosby, 1982.

Lashford, Stephanie. *The Twelve Month Pregnancy. Your Diet From Pre-conception to Motherhood*. Bath, England: Ashgrove Press, 1985.

Liley, A. William. "The Fetus as a Personality." *Australian and New Zealand Journal of Psychiatry* 6 (2), pp. 99-105.

McKay, Susan. *Assertive Childbirth*. Englewood Cliffs, NJ: Prentice-Hall, 1983.

Milinaire, Caterine. *Birth*. New York: Harmony Books, 1971.

Montagu, Ashley. *Life Before Birth*. New York: New American Library, 1964.

Nilsson, Lennart. *The Miracle of Life* (film). Boston: WBGH Educational Foundation, 1983.

Nilsson, Lennart, Axel Ingelman, et al. *A Child is Born*. New York: revised edition, Delacorte, 1977.

Noble, Elizabeth. *Essential Exercises for the Childbearing Year*. Boston, MA: Houghton Mifflin, 1976.

Odent, Michel. *Birth Reborn*. New York: Marion Boyers, 1984.

_____. *Primal Health*. London: Century, 1986.

Pearce, Joseph Chilton. *Exploring the Crack in the Cosmic Egg*. New York: Julian Press, 1974.

Parent Action for Parent Power. 230 N. Michigan Avenue, Suite 1625, Chicago, Illinois 60601.

Petty, Roy. *Home Birth: A Complete Authoritative Guide to the Back-to Basics Trend in Childbirth*. Northbrook, IL: Domus Books, 1989.

Rosen, Mortimer G., and Lynn Rosen. *Your Baby's Brain Before Birth*. New York: New American Library, 1975.

Rugh, Roberts and Landrum Shettles. *From Conception to Birth: The Drama of Life's Beginnings*. New York: Harper & Row, 1971.

Schwartz, Leni. *The Environment of Birth*. Ph.D. Dissertation and Video Tapes. The Union Institute, 1974, Cleveland, Ohio.

_____. *The World of the Unborn*. New York: Marek, 1980.

Sussman, John R., M.D., Levitt B. Blake. *Before You Conceive. The Complete Pregnancy Guide*. New York: Bantam, 1989.

Verny, Thomas, ed. *Pre and Perinatal Psychology: An Introduction*. New York: Human Sciences Press, 1987.

Creative Sex During Pregnancy

Bing, Elisabeth and Libby Colman. *Making Love During Pregnancy*. New York: Bantam, 1977.

Comfort, Alex. *The Joy of Sex*. New York: Crown, 1972.

Gillico, Jerry. *Transcendental Sex: A Meditational Approach to Increasing Sensual Pleasure*. Toronto: Holt, Rinehart & Winston, 1978.

Sources for Growth and Group Work

Anderson, Marianne S., and Louis M. Savary. *Passages: A Guide for Pilgrims of the Mind*. New York: Harper & Row, 1972.

Assagioli, Roberto. *Psychosynthesis*. New York: Viking/Compass, 1965.

Berne, Eric. *Games People Play*. New York: Grove Press, 1969.

Bonny, Helen, and Louis M. Savary. *Music and Your Mind*. New York: Harper & Row, 1973.

Brooks, Charles V. W. *Sensory Awareness: The Rediscovery of Experiencing*. New York: Viking, 1974.

Carter, Mildred. *Helping Yourself With Foot Reflexology*. Englewood Cliffs, NH: Parker, 1969.

Delancey, Gayle. *Living Your Dreams*. New York: Harper & Row, 1979.

Downing, George. *The Massage Book*. New York: Random House, 1974.

Faraday, Ann. *Dream Power*. New York: Coward-McCann, 1972.

Furth, Gregg M. *The Secret World of Drawings: Healing Through Art*. Boston, MA: Sigo Press, 1990.

Garfield, Patricia. *Creative Dreaming*. New York: Simon & Schuster, 1975.

Grossman, Richard. *Choosing and Changing*. New York: E.P. Dutton, 1978.

Gunther, Bernard. *Sense Relaxation*. New York: Collier Books, 1968.

Hannah, Barbara. *Encounters With the Soul: Active Imagination*. Boston: Sigo Press, 1990.

Hills, Christopher, and Deborah Rozman. *Exploring Inner Space: Awareness Games for all Ages*. Boulder Creek, CA: University of Trees, 1978.

Jacobson, Edmund. *Progressive Relaxation*. Chicago: University of Chicago Press, 1974.

_____. *How to Relax and Have Your Baby*. New York: McGraw-Hill, 1959.

Jones, Carl. *Visualizations for an Easier Childbirth*. New York: Simon & Schuster, 1988.

Keyes, Margaret F. *The Inward Journey: Art as Therapy for You*. Millbrae, CA: Celestial ARts, 1974.

Leedy, Jack J. *Poetry, the Healer*. New York: Lippincott, 1973.

Lewis, Howard R., and Dr. Harold S. Streitfeld. *Growth Games*. New York: Harcourt Brace Jovanovich, 1970.

Masters, Robert, and Jean Houston. *Mind Games*. New York: Dell, 1972.

Mindell, Arnold. *Dreambody: The Body's Role in Revealing the Self*. Boston: Sigo Press, 1990.

Nicholl, Maurice. *Dream Psychology*. Boston: Sigo Press, 1990.

Perls, Fritz. *Gestalt Therapy Verbatim*. Lafayette, CA: Real People Press, 1969.

Perls, Fritz, R. Hefferline and P. Goodman. *Gestalt Therapy*. New York: Delta, 1951.

Progoff, Ira. *At a Journal Workshop*. New York: Dialogue House Library, 1975.

Rhyne, Janie. *The Gestalt Art Experience*. Monterey, CA: Brooks/Cole, 1973.

Rogers, Carl R. *On Becoming a Person*. Boston: Houghton Mifflin, 1961.

_____. *On Encounter Groups*. New York: Harper & Row, 1970.

_____. *On Personal Power*. New York: Delacorte, 1977.

Samuels, Mike, and Nancy Samuels. *Seeing With the Mind's Eye*. New York: Random House/Bookworks, 1975.

Satir, Virginia. *Peoplemaking*. Palo Alto, CA: Science & Behavior Books, 1972.

Schultz, William C. *Joy*. New York: Grove Press, 1967.

Simon, Sid. *Caring, Feeling, Touching*. Niles, IL: Argus, 1976.

Smith, David. *The East-WEst Exercise Book*. New York: McGraw-Hill, 1976.

Stevens, John O. *Awareness: Exploring, Experimenting*. New York: Bantam, 1973.

Trungpa, Chogyam. *Dharmas Without Blame*. Berkeley, CA: Shambala Publications, 1973.

Tulku, Tarthang. *Gesture of Balance: A Guide to Awareness, Self-healing and Meditation*. Emeryville, CA: Dharma Publishing, 1977.

_____. *Time, Space and Knowledge: A New Vision of REality*. Emeryville, CA: Dharma Publishing, 1977.

Vaughn, Frances E. *Awakening Intuition*. New York: Anchor Books, 1979.

White, John, and James Fadiman, eds. *Relax: How You Feel Can Feel Better*. New York: Dell, 1976.

Sigo Press also has available an audio tape by Leni Schwartz. It includes several meditations and exercises, similar to those in this book, to use to bond before birth. Running time approximately 60 minutes.